BEHAVIORAL ASSESSMENT AND MANAGEMENT OF CARDIOVASCULAR DISORDERS

Edited by

David S. Krantz, PhD
Uniformed Services University of the Health Sciences

and

James A. Blumenthal, PhD
Duke University Medical Center

Professional Resource Exchange, Inc.
Sarasota, Florida

Copyright © 1987 Professional Resource Exchange, Inc.
Professional Resource Exchange, Inc.
635 South Orange Avenue, Suites 4-6
Post Office Box 15560
Sarasota, FL 34277-1560

All rights reserved

No part of this book may be reproduced, stored in a retrieval system, or transmitted, in any form or by any means, either electronic, mechanical, photocopying, microfilming, recording, or otherwise, without written permission from the publisher.

Printed in the United States of America

ISBN: 0-943158-20-6
Library of Congress Catalog Number: 87-42554

The proofreader for this book was Janet Nunez, the production supervisor was Debbie Fink, the graphics coordinator was Carol Hirsch, the typist was Lois Hartz, the cover designer was Bill Tabler, and the printer was Edwards Brothers, Inc.

Portions of this book originally appeared in the *Journal of Cardiopulmonary Rehabilitation*, special issues on "Stress Management in Health and Rehabilitation": Part I and Part II, May 20, 1985, Vol. V, No. 5 and June 20, 1985, Vol. V, No. 6. The permission of Le Jacq Publishing, Inc. to include that material in this book is gratefully acknowledged.

This book is dedicated to Pauline K. Blustein, Sylvia Ryback, and our parents, Robert and Beatrice Krantz and Ruth Blumenthal.

DSK and JAB

Preface

It is now widely recognized that psychological and behavioral factors are relevant to all aspects of cardiovascular disorders, ranging from etiology to treatment and rehabilitation. Although behavioral science techniques and knowledge are often unfamiliar to medical practitioners, personnel involved in the treatment of cardiac patients must grapple with what are essentially behavioral problems. Such problems include smoking cessation, exercise and medication compliance, dietary management, modification of Type A behavior, and other forms of stress management. Behavioral medicine, an interdisciplinary field of research and practice integrating behavioral science and biomedical knowledge, therefore has much to offer in the treatment of cardiovascular disorders.

Eight out of the ten chapters in this volume were originally prepared for a special issue of the *Journal of Cardiopulmonary Rehabilitation*, guest edited by David Krantz. This special issue was invited to provide the readership of the *Journal* (predominantly practicing cardiologists, exercise physiologists, and nurses) with state-of-the-art information on the importance of problems related to emotional stress for the cardiac patient.

This volume was assembled to present information on biobehavioral approaches to treatment of cardiovascular disorders to psychologists, psychiatrists, and other behavioral science health professionals who may wish to learn about this growing area. Two additional chapters were added to the original eight to provide necessary background information for the behavioral science audience, and to set the other chapters in broader context. These included an introduction and overview of behavior-

Preface

al medicine in the secondary prevention of coronary disease (Chapter 1), and a chapter on the rationale and organization of cardiac rehabilitation programs (Chapter 10).

Authors were asked, in writing each contribution, to make them scholarly and well-grounded scientifically, yet oriented to concerns of the practitioner. Therefore, most of the pieces present basic techniques and their scientific background, and together cover a broad range of behavioral management problems and approaches relevant to cardiovascular disease.

The chapters that follow provide a critical but practical overview of behavioral medicine contributions to the treatment of cardiovascular disease. It is hoped that they will stimulate further research, applications to clinical practice, and understanding of the pervasive influence of psychological and behavioral factors in health promotion and disease prevention and treatment.

As noted previously, portions of this book originally appeared in the *Journal of Cardiopulmonary Rehabilitation*, special issue on "Stress Management in Health and Rehabilitation": Part I and Part II, May 20, 1985, Vol. V, No. 5 and June 20, 1985, Vol. V, No. 6.

The permission of Le Jacq Publishing, Inc. to include that material in this book is gratefully acknowledged.

David S. Krantz
and
James A. Blumenthal

Bethesda, MD and Durham, NC
March, 1987

Table of Contents

PREFACE   v

CONTRIBUTING AUTHORS   ix

1. BEHAVIORAL MEDICINE IN THE SECONDARY PREVENTION OF CARDIOVASCULAR DISEASE: AN OVERVIEW
   James A. Blumenthal and David S. Krantz   1

2. PSYCHOLOGIC ASSESSMENT IN CARDIAC REHABILITATION
   James A. Blumenthal   21

3. COPING WITH THE SEQUELAE OF SMOKING CESSATION
   Neil E. Grunberg and Deborah J. Bowen   41

4. THE PSYCHOLOGIC EFFECTS OF EXERCISE
   Donald Goff and Joel E. Dimsdale   53

5. PSYCHIATRIC MANAGEMENT OF THE HOSPITALIZED CARDIAC PATIENT
   George E. Tesar and Thomas P. Hackett   67

6. BIOBEHAVIORAL TREATMENT APPROACHES FOR CARDIOVASCULAR DISORDERS
   Margaret A. Chesney and Marcia M. Ward   81

Table of Contents

7. ALTERING THE TYPE A
   BEHAVIOR PATTERN IN
   POST-INFARCTION PATIENTS
   *Carl E. Thoresen, Meyer Friedman, Lynda H.
   Powell, James J. Gill, and Diane Ulmer*   97

8. BEHAVIORAL EFFECTS OF BETA
   BLOCKERS: REDUCTION OF ANXIETY,
   ACUTE STRESS, AND TYPE A BEHAVIOR
   *Lynn A. Durel, David S. Krantz,
   John F. Eisold, and Jeffrey D. Lazar*   117

9. PSYCHOLOGIC AND SOCIAL
   OUTCOMES FOLLOWING CORONARY
   ARTERY BYPASS SURGERY
   Julaine Kinchla and Theodore Weiss   133

10. ORGANIZATIONAL AND
    ADMINISTRATIVE OVERVIEW OF
    CARDIAC REHABILITATION PROGRAMS
    Paul M. Ribisl   155

INDEX   175

Contributing Authors

James A. Blumenthal, PhD, is Associate Professor of Psychiatry, Assistant Professor of Medicine, and Senior Fellow, Center for the Study of Aging and Development at Duke University Medical Center, Durham, North Carolina. His research interests are in behavioral approaches to primary and secondary prevention of coronary disease.

Deborah J. Bowen, PhD, is a psychologist on the faculty at the Fred Hutchinson Cancer Research Center, Seattle, Washington, where she conducts research in the area of cancer prevention.

Margaret A. Chesney, PhD, is Director of the Department of Behavioral Medicine at SRI International in Menlo Park, California. Her research interests are in psychosocial factors in hypertension and coronary heart disease.

Joel E. Dimsdale, MD, is Associate Professor of Psychiatry, and Director of the Program in Consultation-Liaison Psychiatry and Behavioral Medicine at the University of California, San Diego. His research interests are in neuroendocrine responses to stress.

Lynn A. Durel, PhD, is Assistant Professor of Psychology at the University of Miami in Coral Gables, Florida. Her research interests concern behavioral effects of beta-blockers, and behavioral pharmacology.

John F. Eisold, MD, is a Lieutenant Commander in the U.S. Navy Medical Corps and Assistant Professor of Medicine at the Uniformed Services University of the Health Sciences, Bethesda, Maryland. He was formerly Chief of the Hypertension Clinic at the Naval Hospital, Bethesda, MD. His interest is in general internal medicine.

Contributing Authors

Meyer Friedman, MD, is a cardiologist who has been doing research in cardiology for 35 years with numerous scientific publications and books to his credit. He is the Director Emeritus of the Harold Brunn Institute of Research at Mt. Zion Hospital in San Francisco and was the Project Director of the Recurrent Coronary Prevention Project. At present he is an honorary member of the Board of Directors and consultant to the Meyer Friedman Institute. He has co-authored two books for the lay public - *Type A Behavior and Your Heart* and *Treating Type A Behavior and Your Heart*.

James J. Gill, MD, is an Associate Professor at Harvard University Health Services, Boston, Massachusetts, and a lecturer in the Social Relations Department. His area of interest is humanistic medicine.

Donald Goff, MD, is Assistant Professor of Psychiatry at Tufts University School of Medicine, Boston, Massachusetts.

Neil E. Grunberg, PhD, is Associate Professor of Medical Psychology at the Uniformed Services University of the Health Sciences, Bethesda, Maryland. His research deals with behavioral and biological effects of cigarette smoking and nicotine.

Thomas P. Hackett, MD, is an Eben S. Draper Professor of Psychiatry at Harvard Medical School, Boston, Massachusetts. He also serves as the Psychiatrist-in-Chief at Massachusetts General Hospital. His research and clinical interests are in the psychology of coronary heart disease and general psychiatry.

Julaine Kinchla, PhD, is in private practice in Princeton, New Jersey, and has an appointment as Associate in Psychiatry at the University of Pennsylvania Medical Center, where she serves as a consultant to the Institute for Cognitive and Behavioral Therapies. She has a special interest in the treatment of weight disorders and in management of Type A behavior patterns.

David S. Krantz, PhD, is Associate Professor of Medical Psychology at Uniformed Services University of the Health Sciences in Bethesda, Maryland. His research interests are in behavioral factors, stress, and cardiovascular disorders. He is currently studying the role of biobehavioral factors in silent myocardial ischemia.

Jeffrey D. Lazar, MD, PhD, is Director of Clinical Pharmacology for Pfizer Central Research, Groton, Connecticut and Associate Professor of Medicine at

Contributing Authors

Brown University School of Medicine. His primary area of expertise is clinical pharmacology.

Lynda H. Powell, PhD, is an Associate Professor of Epidemiology and Public Health at Yale University, School of Medicine, New Haven, Connecticut. Her interests include chronic disease epidemiology and the connection between behavior and coronary heart disease.

Paul M. Ribisl, PhD, is Professor of Health and Sport Science and the Program Director of the Cardiac Rehabilitation Program at Wake Forest University in Winston-Salem, North Carolina. He currently serves as Chairman of the Preventive and Rehabilitative Programs Committee of the American College of Sports Medicine. His interests are in the principles of exercise prescription and standards of care in preventive and rehabilitative programs.

George E. Tesar, MD, is a Clinical Assistant in Psychiatry at Massachusetts General Hospital, Boston, Massachusetts, and Instructor in Psychiatry at Harvard Medical School. His academic interests are in the area of pathophysiology and treatment of anxiety disorders and the interface between cardiology and psychiatry.

Carl E. Thoresen, PhD, is Professor of Education at Stanford University, Palo Alto, California, directing the newly established PhD specialty program in health psychology. He also is Director of Training and Research for the Meyer Friedman Institute, Mt. Zion Hospital, San Francisco. He is interested in psychosocial perspectives on health and disease, including obesity and coronary prone behavior pattern (Type A).

Diane Ulmer, RN, MS, is a nurse researcher with a background in emergency and cardiovascular nursing. Her professional interests are in the area of behavioral medicine, particularly cardiology. She was the Project Supervisor and Field Director for the Recurrent Coronary Prevention Project. At present she is the Executive Director of the Meyer Friedman Institute, San Francisco, California, and has co-authored the book *Treating Type A Behavior and Your Heart*.

Marcia M. Ward, PhD, is Senior Research Psychologist in the Department of Behavioral Medicine at SRI International in Menlo Park, California. She conducts

Contributing Authors

research on psychophysiological correlates of hypertension and coronary heart disease.

Theodore Weiss, MD, is Clinical Associate Professor of Psychiatry at the University of Pennsylvania, and a member of the psychiatry departments at Presbyterian-University of Pennsylvania Medical Center and Lankenau Hospital in Philadelphia. He has a longstanding interest in the psychiatry-cardiology interface.

BEHAVIORAL ASSESSMENT
AND
MANAGEMENT
OF
CARDIOVASCULAR DISORDERS

Behavioral Medicine in the Secondary Prevention of Cardiovascular Disease: An Overview*

James A. Blumenthal and David S. Krantz

It has become apparent that traditional biomedical approaches to health care have important limitations when applied to the prevention and rehabilitation of patients with coronary heart disease (CHD). Despite recent declines in CHD mortality, diseases of the cardiovascular system remain the single most prevalent cause of death in the United States.[1] Thousands of Americans suffer myocardial infarctions each day, incurring an estimated total economic cost in excess of $60 billion annually.[2] Although advances in surgical and medical treatment have probably contributed to the declining death rates from CHD in the United States, changes in lifestyle factors related to coronary risk are also considered important.

People who are sedentary, smoke, overeat, exhibit Type A behavior, and experience high levels of psychological stress are at risk for the development of CHD and are at greater risk for subsequent morbidity and mortality. Thus, specialists in cardiac rehabilitation have recognized the importance of *behavior* in the etiology and treatment of CHD.

---

*Preparation of this article was supported, in part, by grants from the NIH - HL31514, HL30675, AG04238, and by a grant from the John D. and Catherine T. MacArthur Foundation. Also, portions of this article were adapted from Cardiac rehabilitation: A new frontier for behavioral medicine, Journal of Cardiac Rehabilitation 1983;3(9):637-656.

Behavioral medicine is defined as "the interdisciplinary field concerned with the development and integration of behavioral and biomedical science knowledge and techniques relevant to health and illness, and the application of these techniques to prevention, diagnosis, treatment, and rehabilitation."[3] Interest in the relationship between behavior and heart disease is not new. In one of the earliest descriptions of a relationship between behavioral characteristics and CHD, Osler[4] noted that the potential coronary-prone individual was "the keen and ambitious man, the indicator of whose engines are set full speed ahead." Franz Alexander,[5] followed by subsequent psychosomatic researchers, developed a theory that emotional conflicts could cause specific organic diseases as a result of prolonged autonomic arousal. For example, chronic inhibited aggressive impulses associated with anxiety and fear were hypothesized to play an etiologic role in the development of arterial hypertension.

By the 1960s, however, the lack of progress in developing effective treatment techniques, the theoretical preoccupation with psychodynamic concepts, and the lack of experimentally-oriented data prompted many researchers and practitioners to reconceptualize their theoretical and therapeutic approaches to the treatment of patients with CHD. The emergence of modern behaviorism[6] and the success of behavior modification and behavior therapy for the treatment of maladaptive behaviors served to attract many professionals concerned with treatment.

Since CHD is such a significant health problem in this country, understanding the role that environmental and behavioral factors play in the pathogenesis of CHD is a major challenge, as well as an opportunity for behavioral scientists. In recognition of the importance of behavioral factors, efforts to treat patients with established coronary disease have recently expanded beyond pharmacological and surgical approaches to include such strategies as diet modification, exercise, stress management, Type A behavior modification, weight reduction, smoking cessation, and methods to enhance compliance with various prescribed medical therapies (see, for example, Chapter 10). The chapters in this volume highlight progress in several of these important areas. In this introductory chapter, we will overview current knowledge in the area of secondary prevention of coronary disease, and provide an introduction to the topics covered in this volume. In Chapter 2, Blumenthal underscores the psychological as well as physical impact of CHD and outlines a comprehensive assessment plan for patients in secondary prevention programs.

Secondary prevention of CHD is a term used to describe therapeutic efforts in patients with established coronary disease. In general, those risk factors that are predictive of initial coronary events appear to be less important once the disease has developed. For example, information has been gathered on over 2,000 medically treated patients with coronary artery disease documented by coronary angiography at Duke University Medical Center. No significant independent statistical relationship was found among such traditional risk factors as serum cholesterol, systolic or diastolic blood pressure, or presence of diabetes at the time of cardiac catheterization and subsequent mortality. Similarly, it has been reported[7] that traditional risk factors were only weakly related to subsequent mortality in patients after heart attack, or myocardial infarction (MI). Therefore, it is important to note that efforts to prevent secondary CHD events may have limited success if based solely on the rationale for preventing initial events.

Traditionally, the effectiveness of secondary prevention has been measured by cardiovascular morbidity, especially reinfarction, and mortality. The efficacy of behavioral treatments in affecting these clinical end points will be considered along with other potentially relevant outcomes, especially improvements in quality of life.

SMOKING

The benefits of not smoking have been established in numerous prospective and retrospective studies and are usually inferred from the reduction in morbidity and mortality in ex-smokers relative to those who maintained their smoking habit.[8-12] Several studies have attempted to assess the benefits of smoking discontinuation in patients with established coronary disease. Sparrow and co-workers,[11] for example, found an 18.8% mortality 6 years after a documented MI in a group of men who subsequently stopped smoking, compared to a 30.4% mortality in smokers who maintained their smoking habit or resumed smoking after their infarctions. This reduced risk of death among post-MI patients who stop smoking is consistent with data from other studies in the United States,[13] Sweden,[14] and Ireland.[15] However, these studies report rates based upon spontaneous quitting, and do not evaluate the impact of treatment programs.

The literature on smoking cessation programs has received extensive review,[16-21] and is summarized in Chapter 3 by Grunberg and Bowen. In general, no one method or procedure appears more effective than any other, although certain behavioral techniques are widely employed in most programs. Programs emphasizing nicotine fading (brand switching), controlled smoking (e.g., "take shorter puffs"), chewing nicotine gum, and such self-control procedures as relaxation training and contingency management are widely used, although no study has reported their efficacy in cardiac rehabilitation. Although rapid smoking is the most popular aversive technique, it may have potentially harmful side effects in patients with known CHD.[22,23] Other techniques such as focused smoking[24] or smoke holding[25] may be particularly appropriate for cardiac patients.

Smoking cessation programs need not be complicated and expensive to be effective. For example, several studies have shown that smoking cessation can be achieved by mail[26] or television messages.[27,28] In a systematic study by Jeffrey and colleagues[29] using correspondence (mail) and various combinations of behavioral contracts, follow-up telephone calls, and homework assignments, between 33% and 44% of subjects reported that they were abstinent at 8 months. However, attrition rates are generally high, and there has not been an evaluation of the effectiveness of such procedures in cardiac patient populations. The use of cognitive-behavioral relapse prevention programs has been shown to improve maintenance of desired behavior change. However, few studies have looked at long-term abstinence rates, and no study has considered coronary patients as the specific focus for evaluating the efficacy of the intervention. Grunberg and Bowen focus on techniques for coping with the difficulties of smoking cessation in Chapter 3.

DIET AND WEIGHT CONTROL

Traditionally, patients with coronary disease are encouraged to alter their usual diets. The rationale is largely based on the association between cholesterol, diet, and subsequent mortality in populations initially free of overt CHD such as those studied in Framingham[30] and Chicago.[31]

Reductions in salt intake, cholesterol, and total caloric consumption are routinely suggested in most cardiac rehabilitation settings. (See Chapter 10 by Ribisl.) The aims of dietary treatment include: (a) reduction of elevated plasma cholesterol and triglycerides, (b) maintenance of normal blood pressure, and (c) total reduction of body weight. Although a variety of diets has been proposed, the "alternative diet"[32] or one of its variants is most often recommended for treatment of hyperlipidemia. Basically, this diet recommends reduction of cholesterol intake to 100 mg/day, dietary fat to 20% of total calories, and meat consumption to 84-112 g (3-4 oz)/day, and encourages the exclusive use of low-cholesterol cheeses. However, despite the evidence that dietary intake of salt, saturated fat, and cholesterol play a role in the pathogenesis of coronary atherosclerosis and hypertension,[33-35] no definitive evidence exists that modification of diet has any significant impact on the morbidity or mortality of patients with coronary disease, despite clinical evidence that weight loss can significantly reduce plasma lipid levels.[36,37] Although there is some suggestion that dietary management may lead to regression of atheromatous lesions in humans as well as in animals,[38] these data are far too limited to draw any definitive conclusions in humans.

The effectiveness of behavioral treatments of hyperlipidemia has been recently reviewed.[39] Three controlled clinical trials of diet modification in high-risk adults[40-42] and in normal male volunteers[43] have recently been published. Results of both the National Diet-Heart and Lipid Research studies demonstrated that initial habit changes and resulting reductions in lipid levels could be achieved, although these improvements were not maintained over extended follow-up periods.

Weight loss is usually considered the yardstick of success for any diet program. Assessment of obesity is, therefore, critical. In a recent review of the literature, Brownell[44] has noted the problems of relying solely upon self-report data. He suggests combining multiple measures of obesity, including assessments of body fat (skinfold calipers), absolute body weight, percentage overweight, and body mass index (weight/height^2).

Numerous studies have evaluated the effectiveness of different programs in treating obesity. Several studies have compared the efficacy of behavioral programs with more traditional diet programs.[45-48] In general, behavioral programs appear to be superior, at least in terms of short-term effects.[49,50] It has been noted that most behavioral programs are relatively comparable, with the largest improvements in programs using self-management techniques such as self-monitoring, stimulus control, contingency contracting, exercise, and appetite suppressants. As in the smoking cessation literature, however, there are virtually no controlled studies on the behavioral treatment of obesity in cardiac populations. Moreover, most studies have methodologic limitations (e.g., limited sample sizes, exclusive use of college students, sole reliance on mildly obese subjects, failure to report dropout rates, etc.) that make it difficult to interpret the results. Furthermore, the success of behavioral treatments in maintaining significant weight loss has not been consistently demonstrated. For example, only 2 of 19 recently reviewed studies reported follow-up periods of more than 6 months,[51] and the problems of high recidivism rates in programs that are successful in achieving initial weight loss should not be underestimated.[52]

PHYSICAL EXERCISE TRAINING

There is currently a great deal of interest in the role of physical conditioning in the rehabilitation of the coronary patient. Numerous reviews are available to the interested reader.[53-59] Chapter 4 in this volume by Goff and Dimsdale reviews psychologic benefits of exercise.

In addition to the physiologic effects of exercise, other beneficial effects include a reduction in risk factors such as weight, serum triglycerides, cholesterol and free fatty acids, and improved glucose tolerance,[60,61] as well as psychologic effects (see Goff and Dimsdale, Chapter 4, and Ribisl, Chapter 10). Several studies have demonstrated that angina does not occur until higher double or triple products (i.e., heart rate X blood pressure) are reached, thus suggesting increased myocardial oxygen consumption (and presumably increased coronary blood flow) prior to the onset of ischemia.[62] Although even patients with poor cardiac function can achieve significant improvements in functional capacity,[63] the relative contributions of peripheral circulatory adaptations and improved myocardial function in producing increased exercise capacity in coronary patients appear to vary among individual patients. Some patients can increase exercise capacity without change in indices of cardiac performance, whereas other patients demonstrate increased cardiac performance after a period of exercise training.

Despite the improved cardiovascular fitness and reduction in risk factors as a result of exercise training, evidence for prolongation of life or a reduction in reinfarction in patients with documented CHD remains equivocal. Several studies have reported lowered morbidity among patients who engage in regular exercise,[64,65,66] although methodologic problems and relatively small differences between exercise groups and controls have left the issue unsettled. For example, in the National Exercise and Heart Disease program,[67] the cumulative 3-year total mortality rate was 7.3% for the control group and 4.6% for the exercise group. The 3-year rate for recurrent infarctions was 7.0% and 5.3% for control and exercise groups, respectively. Kellerman[66] studied patients who participated in brief (4-month) and extended (12-42-month) exercise programs. Mortality was lowest in the extended group, and no significant difference was observed between the brief group and no-exercise controls. These findings suggest that benefits of exercise may be achieved only by continued maintenance of the exercise regimen. Studies with high dropout rates also showed no differences in morbidity or mortality between exercise groups and controls,[64,65] suggesting the need for compliance with exercise prescriptions in order to induce clinically significant benefits.

The problem of exercise maintenance has been recently reviewed.[68] As in the previous discussions on smoking and diet, the problem of high attrition rates is a major obstacle limiting the effectiveness of the treatment. However, there has been considerable literature on exercise compliance in cardiac rehabilitation, at least in terms of identifying individuals at risk for noncompliance in cardiac rehabilitation, and for categorizing situational determinants of poor compliance. Unfortunately, behavioral strategies designed to enhance compliance with exercise in cardiac rehabilitation programs have not been implemented. The general problem of noncompliance will be given special consideration in a later section of this review.

TYPE A BEHAVIOR PATTERN

The Type A behavior pattern refers to a constellation of psychologic traits, overt behaviors, and response tendencies. (See Chapter 7 by Thoresen, Friedman, Powell, Gill, and Ulmer). Type A individuals are hard-driving, competitive, aggressive, and impatient. In contrast, Type B individuals are characterized by a relative absence of these characteristics. In retrospective and prospective studies,[69] the Type A behavior pattern is associated with over twice the rate of new coronary events compared to the Type B behavior pattern.*

Recently, specific attempts have been made to alter risk factors for coronary disease in Type A individuals. These efforts are reviewed in Chapter 7 by Thoresen et al and need not be detailed here. Suffice it to say, behavioral strategies have been shown to be effective in reducing Type A behavior, and such reductions may be associated with lowered rates of morbidity and cardiac mortality.

PSYCHOSOCIAL AND OTHER BEHAVIORAL INTERVENTIONS

Although a rather extensive literature has developed on the psychological, social, and behavioral aspects of coronary disease,[70,71] the number of psychologic intervention studies in patients with CHD is fairly limited (see chapters by Chesney and Ward, Tesar and Hackett, and Kinchla and Weiss). Several studies suggest that psychological treatment can facilitate early return to work,[72] reduce emotional disturbance,[73,74,76] increase cardiovascular functioning,[75] and minimize post-infarction complications.[80,82] Psychologic approaches to intervention with coronary patients in both acute and post-hospital phases of illness are given considerable attention in this volume.

The use of biofeedback has also been recently employed in the treatment of cardiac disorders (see Chesney

---

*Recent studies have reported inconsistent associations between Type A behavior and manifestations of CHD. (See Matthews & Haynes[101] for review.) However, components of Type A behavior, such as hostility, have been related to CHD in this research.

and Ward, Chapter 6). Cardiac arrhythmias, particularly those characterized by premature ventricular contractions (PVCs), have been shown to be reduced by employing biofeedback of heart rate responses.[77] For example, Weiss and Engel[78] were able to demonstrate a reduction in the presence of PVCs in four of eight patients treated by heart rate feedback. Other investigators have also reported successful outcomes using biofeedback for PVCs,[79-81] sinus tachycardia,[82,83] and cardiac neurosis[84] (see Chapter 6).

There has also been renewed understanding of the psychologic and psychiatric issues confronting the coronary patient who is coping with the acute phase of illness. These issues are reviewed in Chapter 5 by Tesar and Hackett.

COMPLIANCE WITH MEDICAL REGIMENS

The problem of noncompliance represents a major obstacle to providing effective medical care in patients with coronary disease. The importance of compliance was recently demonstrated when it was suggested that patients who comply with any treatment may have a lower incidence of cardiac events, even if the treatment is a placebo.[85] In one report of the factors influencing prognosis following MI, compliance was the most important single determinant of subsequent fatal and nonfatal reinfarction.[86] In addition, a recent study of determinants of sudden death during exercise in a cardiac rehabilitation program also found the most important factors to be the failure to comply with heart rate restrictions and the presence of silent myocardial ischemia with exercise.[87]

Compliance behavior may be defined as the extent to which the patient's behavior coincides with clinical prescription. Compliant behavior encompasses a variety of behaviors including the taking of medication, following diets, changing activities, or making other lifestyle adjustments such as exercising or smoking cessation, following-up on referrals, and keeping appointments. Although the frequency of noncompliant behavior varies considerably among studies, depending on the kind of problem and the kinds of behavioral adjustments required, the strikingly high number of patients who will not adhere to prescribed treatment regimens must be recognized. For example, 50% of patients who begin an exercise program typically discontinue it within the first 6 months;[88] 50% of patients diagnosed as hypertensive during a blood pressure screening will not keep their first appointment;[89] 75% of patients fail to follow physician advice following discharge from the coronary care unit;[90] and as many as 95% of patients who enter weight reduction programs fail to achieve and maintain their desired weight.[91]

An important step in overcoming the dropout problem involves the identification of those factors in both the individual and the environment that contribute to noncompliance. Characteristics of the rehabilitation program, social supports available, and perceptions of the treatment regimen need to be carefully assessed. Among those factors implicated as being most relevant are the complexity and duration of treatment, the degree of behavior change required by the treatment, the patient's perception of his/her vulnerability, and the potential success of treatment contingent upon compliance.[92,93]

Patient comprehension of the treatment program is perhaps most important. For example, it has been shown that more than 17% of patient errors can be corrected simply by reinstruction.[94] Most patients can only remember two-thirds of what they are told after an initial visit.[95,96] Consequently, simple instructions must often be repeated until patients understand the treatment plan and the rationale for its prescription. Second, the greater the degree of behavior change required, the greater the likelihood for noncompliance. The patient who is asked to change many habits (e.g., stop smoking, modify diet, and begin to exercise) is potentially at greatest risk for noncompliance.[97] Leventhal[98] has noted that education for positive health practices must not only provide information about the consequences of disease to enhance patient motivation but must also attend to the behavioral changes required. Finally, the longer the treatment is maintained, the lower the compliance rate will become. For example, the rate of compliance for short-term regimens may be 15% greater than for long-term regimens.

Few systematic efforts to increase compliance behavior in cardiac rehabilitation settings have been published, although studies with other patient populations have clear implications for cardiac rehabilitation. For example, Dunbar and Stunkard[99] have presented a set of strategies to improve compliance, including establishing behavioral contracts, requiring specific assignments, and tailoring the regimen to meet the needs of the individual patient.

The problem of maintenance of behavior change is even more difficult than that of achieving initial behavior change. Continuing support, self-monitoring, and preventing overdependence on the provider may be particularly helpful. Family cooperation, group support, and behavioral self-management techniques appear to be promising. However, few long-term studies evaluating the effects of behavioral interventions on the maintenance of behavior change have been conducted. In their excellent review of compliance with pharmacologic regimens, Epstein and Cluss[100] note that the inconsistent relationship between adherence and clinical outcome may be due to the limitations of the treatment itself. Thus, it will be possible to evaluate more realistically the clinical significance of any given treatment when more effective compliance strategies are developed.

CONCLUSION

There have been significant advances in the treatment of patients with coronary disease. Available evidence indicates decreased rates of reinfarction and death are now being achieved, in part due to advances in pharmacologic treatment, treatments which themselves have measurable psychological effects. (See Chapter 8 by Durel, Krantz, Eisold, and Lazar on psychologic effects of beta-blockers.) However, the traditional concept of secondary prevention should be expanded beyond the exclusive considerations of reinfarction and mortality. Improving the quality of life, including psychologic wellbeing, and increasing the ability to return to work and perform various physical activities are also recognized as important goals of cardiac rehabilitation. (See Kinchla and Weiss, Chapter 9 for discussion of issues in postcoronary bypass surgery recovery.)

A multifaceted program, including smoking cessation, diet modification, exercise, stress management, and Type A behavior modification, is the most prudent approach to secondary prevention at this time. The use of behavioral treatment strategies offers promising results when combined with appropriate medical interventions. In addition, the problem of noncompliance affects all aspects of coronary rehabilitation and should not be overlooked.

REFERENCES

1. National Center for Health Statistics: *Monthly Vital Statistics Report* (DHHS Pub. No. [PHS] 80-1120) Sept. 1980;29:6.
2. *Eighth Report of the Director of the National Heart, Lung, and Blood Institute.* Government Printing Office, Washington, DC, March 1981.
3. Schwartz GE, Weiss SM: Yale Conference on Behavioral Medicine: A proposed definition and statement of goals. *J Behav Med* 1978;1:3-12.
4. Osler W: The Humleian lectures on angina pectoris. *Lancet* 1910;1:3-12.
5. Alexander F: *Psychosomatic Medicine: Its Principles and Applications.* New York, Norton, 1950.
6. Skinner BF: *Science and Human Behavior.* New York, MacMillan, 1953.
7. Coronary Drug Project Research Group: Initial findings leading to modification of its research and protocol. *JAMA* 1970;219:1303.
8. *Smoking and Health: A Report of the Surgeon General,* publication 79-50066. US Department of Health, Education, and Welfare, Public Health Service, 1979.
9. Doll R, Hill AB: Mortality in relation to smoking: Ten years' observations of British doctors. *Br J Med* 1964;1:1460-1467.
10. Hammond EC, Garfinkel L: Coronary heart disease, stroke and aortic aneurysm: Factors in the etiology. *Arch Environ Health* 1969;19:167-182.
11. Sparrow D, Dawber TR, Colson T: The influence of cigarette smoking on prognosis after a first myocardial infarction. *J Chron Diseases* 1978;31:425-432.
12. Friedman GD, Petitti DB, Bawol RD, Siegelaub AB: Mortality in cigarette smokers and quitters: Effect of baseline differences. *N Engl J Med* 1981;304:1407-1410.
13. Coronary Drug Project Research Group: Cigarette smoking as a risk factor in men with a prior history of myocardial infarction. *J Chron Diseases* 1979;32:415-425.
14. Wilhelmsen L, Vedin JA, Elmfeldt D, Tibbin G, Wilhelmssen L: Smoking and myocardial infarction. *Lancet* 1975;1:415-420.
15. Mulcahy R, Hickey N, Graham IM, Macairt J: Factors affecting the five-year survival rate of men following acute coronary heart disease. *Am Heart J* 1977;93:556-559.

16. Schwartz JL: A critical review and evaluation of smoking control methods. *Pub Health Rep* 1969;84:483-506.
17. Bernstein DA: Modification of smoking behavior: An evaluative review. *Psychol Bull* 1969;71:418-440.
18. Leventhal H, Cleary PD: The smoking problem: A review of the research and theory in behavioral risk modification. *Psychol Bull* 1980;88:370-405.
19. Evans RI, Henderson AH, Hill PC, Rains BE: Current psychological, social, and educational programs in control and prevention of smoking: A critical methodological review. *Ather Rev* 1979;6:203.
20. Lichtenstein E, Danaher BG: Modification of smoking A critical analysis of theory, research, and practice, in Hersen M, Eisler RM, Miller PM (eds): *Progress in Behavior Modification*, vol. 3. New York, Academic Press, 1978.
21. Lichtenstein E: The smoking problem: A behavioral perspective. *J Consult Clin Psychol* 1982;50:804-819.
22. Horan JJ, Hackette G, Nicholas WC, Linberg SE, Stone CI, Lukaski HC: Rapid smoking: A cautionary note. *J Consult Clin Psychol* 1977;45:341-343.
23. Hall RG, Sachs DPL, Hall SM: Medical risks and therapeutic effectiveness of rapid smoking. *Behav Ther* 1979;10:249-259.
24. Hackett G, Horan JJ: Focused smoking: An unequivocally safe alternative to rapid smoking. *J Drug Ed* 1978;8:261-265.
25. Kopel SA, Suckerman KR, Baksht A: *Smoke Holding*. Paper presented at the annual meeting of the Association for the Advancement of Behavior Therapy, San Francisco, December 1979.
26. Brengelmann JC: The treatment of smoking through the mail, in Schwartz JC (ed): *Progress in Smoking Cessation*. New York, American Cancer Society, 1978:255-265.
27. Best JA: Mass media, self-management and smoking modification, in Davidson PO, Davidson SM (eds): *Behavioral Medicine: Changing Health Lifestyles*. New York, Brunner/Mazel, 1980.
28. McAlister AL: Mass communication of cessation counseling: Combining television and self-help groups, in Schwartz J (ed): *Progress in Smoking Cessation*. New York, American Cancer Society, 1978:284-287.
29. Jeffrey RW, Danaher BG, Killen J, Farquhar JW, Kinnier R: Self-administered programs for health behavior change: Smoking cessation and weight reduction by mail. *Addict Behav* 1982;7:57-63.

30. Truett J, Cornfield J, Kannel W: A multivariate analysis of the risk of coronary disease. *J Chron Diseases* 1967;20:511-524.
31. Shekelle RB, Shryrock AM, Paul O, Lepper M, Stamler J, Liv S, Raynor WJ: Diet, serum cholesterol, and death from coronary heart disease. *N Engl J Med* 1981; 304:65-70.
32. Connor WE, Connor SL: Dietary treatment of hyperlipidemia, in Rifkind BM, Levy RI (eds): *Hyperlipidemia: Diagnosis and Therapy.* New York, Grune & Stratton, 1977.
33. Epstein F: The epidemiology of coronary heart disease: A review. *J Chron Diseases* 1965;18:735-774.
34. Keys A: The individual risk of coronary heart disease. *Annals of the New York Academy of Science* 1966; 134:1046-1056.
35. Simborg DW: The status of risk factors and coronary heart disease. *J Chron Diseases* 1970;22:515-552.
36. Hall Y, Stamler J, Cohen DB: Effectiveness of a low saturated fat, low cholesterol, weight reducing diet for the control of hypertriglyceridemia. *Atherosclerosis* 1972; 16:384-403.
37. Stamler J, Berkson DM, Lindberg HA: Risk factors: Their role in the etiology and pathogenesis of the atherosclerotic diseases, in Wissler RW, Greer JC (eds): *Pathogenesis of Atherosclerosis.* Baltimore, Williams & Wilkins, 1972.
38. Wissler RW: Nutrition, plasma lipids, and atherosclerosis, in Laver RM, Shekelle RB (eds): *Childhood Prevention of Atherosclerosis and Hypertension.* New York, Raven Press, 1980:94.
39. Carmody TP, Fey SG, Pierce DK, Connor WE, Matarazzo JD: Behavioral treatment of hyperlipidemia: Techniques, results and future directions. *J Behav Med* 1982;5:91-116.
40. Kuller L, Neaton J, Cagginla A, Falvo-Gerald L: Primary prevention of heart attacks: The multiple risk factor intervention trial. *Am J Epid* 1980;112:185-199.
41. Multiple Risk Factor Intervention Trial (MRFIT): A national study of primary prevention of coronary heart disease. *J Med Assoc* 1976;235:249-258.
42. Haback PA, Schrott HG, Connor WE: The coronary primary prevention trial. *J Iowa Med Soc* 1974;64:19-28.
43. National Diet-Heart Study Research Group: The national diet-heart study final report. *Circulation* 1968; 37(suppl 1).

44. Brownell KD: Obesity: Understanding and treating a serious, prevalent, and refractory disorder. *J Consult Clin Psychol* 1982;50:820-840.
45. Meyer AJ, Henderson JB: Multiple risk factor reduction in the prevention of cardiovascular disease. *Preventive Med* 1974;3:225-236.
46. Foreyt, JP, Scott LW, Mitchell RE, Gotto AM: Plasma lipid changes in the normal population following behavioral treatment. *J Consult Clin Psychol* 1979;47:440-452.
47. Meyer AJ, Nash JD, McAlister AL, Maccoby N, Farquhar JW: Skills training in a cardiovascular health education campaign. *J Consult Clin Psychol* 1980;48:129-142.
48. Stern MP, Farquhar JW, Maccoby N, Russell SH: Results of a two-year health education campaign on dietary behavior: The Stanford Three-Community Study. *Circulation* 1976;54:826-833.
49. Stunkard AJ: From explanation to action in psychosomatic medicine: The case of obesity. *Psychosom Med* 1975;37:195-236.
50. Stuart RB: Weight loss and beyond: Are they taking it off and keeping it off? in Davidson PO, Davidson SM (eds): *Behavioral Medicine: Changing Health Lifestyles.* New York, Brunner/Mazel, 1980.
51. Hall SM, Hall RG: Outcome and methodological considerations in behavioral treatment of obesity. *Behav Ther* 1974;5:352-364.
52. Hall SM, Hall RG, DeBoer G, O'Kulitch P: Self and external management compared with psychotherapy in the control of obesity. *Behav Res Therapy* 1977;15:89-95.
53. Haskell WL: Physical activity after myocardial infarction. *Am J Cardiology* 1974;33:776.
54. Bruce RA: The benefits of physical training for patients with coronary heart disease, in Gelfinger FJ, Elbert RV, Finland M, Relman AS (eds): *Controversy in Internal Medicine.* Philadelphia, W. B. Saunders, 1974.
55. Amsterdam EA, Wilmore JH, DeMaria AN: *Exercise in Cardiovascular Health and Disease.* New York, Yorke Medical Books, 1977.
56. Mitchell JH: Exercise training in the treatment of coronary heart disease. *Adv Int Med* 1975;20:249-272.
57. Froelicher VF: Does exercise conditioning delay progression of myocardial ischemia in coronary atherosclerotic heart disease. *Cardiovascular Clinician* 1977;8:11-31.
58. Scheur J, Tipton CM: Cardiovascular adjustments to physical training. *Annual Rev of Physiol* 1977;39:221-251.

59. Greenberg MA, Arbeit S, Rubin IL: The role of physical training in patients with coronary artery disease. *Am Heart J* 1979;97:527-534.

60. Clausen JP, Larsen OA, Trap-Jensen J: Physical training in the management of coronary artery disease. *Circulation* 1969;40:143-154.

61. Bjernulf A, Boberg J, Froberg S: Physical training after myocardial infarction: Metabolic effects during short and prolonged exercise before and after physical training in male patients after myocardial infarction. *Scand J of Clin Lab Investi* 1975;33:173-185.

62. Redwood DR, Rosing DR, Epstein SE: Circulatory and symptomatic effects of physical training in patients with coronary artery disease and angina pectoris. *N Engl J Med* 1972;286:959-965.

63. Conn EH, Williams RS, Wallace AG: Exercise responses before and after physical conditioning in patients with severely depressed left ventricular function. *Am J Cardiology* 1982;49:296-300.

64. Kentala E; Physical fitness and feasibility of physical rehabilitation after myocardial infarction in men of working age. *Annals of Clin Res* 1972;9(suppl):1-84.

65. Wilhelmsen L, Sanne H, Elmfeldt D, Grimby G, Tibblin G, Wedel H: A controlled trial of physical training after myocardial infarction. *Prevent Med* 1975;4:491-508.

66. Kellerman JJ: Physical conditioning in patients after myocardial infarction: Results of a comparative study and nine years follow-up. *Schweizerische Medizinische Wochenscrift* 1973;102:79-85.

67. National Exercise and Heart Disease Program. Effects of a prescribed supervised exercise program on mortality and cardiovascular morbidity in patients after a myocardial infarction. *Am J Cardiology* 1981;48:39-46.

68. Dishman RK: Compliance/adherence in health-related exercise. *Health Psychol* 1982;1:237-267.

69. Rosenman RH, Brand RJ, Jenkins CD, Friedman M, Strauss R, Wurm M: Coronary heart disease in the Western Collaborative Group Study: Final follow-up experience of 8 1/2 years. *J Am Med Assoc* 1975;233:872-877.

70. Jenkins CD: Psychologic and social precursors in coronary disease. *N Engl J Med* 1971;284:244-307.

71. Jenkins CD: Recent evidence supporting psychological and social risk factors for coronary disease. *N Engl J Med* 1976;294:987-994,1033-1038.

72. Thockcloth RM, Ho SO, Wright W: Is cardiac rehabilitation really necessary. *Med J Australia* 1973;2:669-674.
73. Adsett CA, Bruhn JG: Short-term group psychotherapy for post-myocardial infarction patients and their wives. *Canadian Med Assoc J* 1968;99:577-584.
74. Gruen W: Effects of brief psychotherapy during the hospitalization period or the recovery process in heart attacks. *J Consult Clin Psychol* 1975;43:223-232.
75. Ornish D, Scherwitz LW, Doody RS, Keston D, McLanahan SM, Brown SE, DePuey EG, Sonnemaker R, Haynes C, Lester J, McAllister GK, Hall RJ, Burdine JA, Gotta AM Jr: Effects of stress management training and dietary changes in treating ischemic heart disease. *J Am Med Assoc* 1983;249:54-59.
76. Rahe RH, O'Neil T, Hagan A, Arthur RJ: Brief group therapy following myocardial infarction: Eighteen-month follow-up of a controlled trial. *Psychiat in Med* 1975;6:349-358.
77. Engel BT, Bleecher ER: Application of operant conditioning techniques to the control of cardiac arrhythmias, in Obrist PA, Black AH, Brener J, DiCara LV (eds): *Cardiovascular Physiology*. Chicago, Aldine Publishing, 1974.
78. Weiss T, Engel BT: Operant conditioning of heart rate in patients with premature ventricular contractions. *Psychosom Med* 1971;33:301-331.
79. Pickering T, Gorham G: Learned heart rate controlled by a patient with ventricular parasystolic rhythm. *Lancet* 1975;1:252-253.
80. Benson H, Alexander S, Feldman CL: Decreased premature ventricular contractions through the use of the relaxation response in patients with stable ischemic heart disease. *Lancet* 1975;2:380-382.
81. Lown B, Temtl JB, Reich P: Basis for recurring ventricular fibrillation in the absence of coronary heart disease and its management. *N Engl J Med* 1976;294:623-629.
82. Blanchard EB, Abel GG: An experimental study of the biofeedback treatment of a rape-induced psychophysiological cardiovascular disorder. *Behav Ther* 1976;7:113-119.
83. Scott RW, Blanchard EB, Edmunson ED, Young LD: A shaping procedure for heart-rate control in chronic tachycardia. *Percept Motor Skills* 1973;37:327-338.
84. Wickramasekera I: Heart rate feedback and the management of cardiac neurosis. *J Abn Psychol* 1974;83:578-580.

85. Coronary Drug Project Research Group: Initial findings leading to modification of its research and protocol. *JAMA* 1970;219:1303.
86. Shephard RJ, Corey P, Kavanaugh T: Exercise compliance and the prevention of a recurrence of myocardial infarction. *Med Sci Sports & Exercise* 1981;13:1-5.
87. Hossack KE, Hartwig R: Cardiac arrest during cardiac rehabilitation: Identification of high risk patients (abstract). *Am J Cardiology* 1982;49:915.
88. Carmody TP, Senner JW, Matinow MR, Matarazzo JD: Physical exercise rehabilitation: Long-term dropout rate in cardiac patients. *J Behav Med* 1980;3:113-168.
89. Finnerty FA, Mattie E, Finnerty FA: Hypertension in the Inner City: I. Analysis of clinic dropouts. *Circulation* 1973;47:73-75.
90. Johnson WL: *Conformity to Medical Recommendations in Coronary Heart Disease*. Paper presented at American Sociology Association Meeting, Chicago, September 1965.
91. Dunbar J, Stunkard A: Adherence to diet and drug regimen, in Levy R, Rifkind B, Dennis B, Ernst N (eds): *Nutrition, Lipids and Coronary Heart Disease*. New York, Raven Press, 1979:391-423.
92. Blackwell B: Treatment adherence. *Br J Psychol* 1976;129:510.
93. Haynes RB: Determinants of compliance: The disease and mechanics of treatment, in Haynes RB, Taylor DW, Sackett DL (eds): *Compliance in Health Care*. Baltimore, Johns Hopkins University Press, 1976.
94. Hulka BS, Cassel JC, Kupper LL: Disparities between medications prescribed and consumed among chronic disease patients, in Lasagna L (ed): *Patient Compliance*. New York, Futura Publishing, 1976:123-152.
95. Joyce CRB, Capla G, Mason M, Reynolds E, Matthews JA: Quantitative study of doctor-patient communication. *J of Med* 1969;38:183.
96. Ley P: Memory for medical information. *Br J Soc Clin Psychol* 1979;18:245.
97. Baile WF, Engel BT: A behavioral strategy for promoting treatment compliance following myocardial infarction, in Franck CM, Wilson GT (eds): *Annual Rev of Behav Ther*. New York, Brunner/Mazel, 1979.
98. Leventhal H: Changing attitudes and habits to reduce risk factors in chronic disease. *Am J Cardiology* 1973;31:571-580.
99. Dunbar JM, Stunkard AJ: Adherence to medical regimens, in Levy R, Rifkind B, Dennis B, Ernst M (eds):

Nutrition, Lipids and Coronary Heart Disease. New York, Raven Press, 1979:391-494.
100. Epstein LH, Cluss PA: A behavioral medicine perspective on adherence to long-term medical regimens. *J Consult Clin Psychol* 1982;50:950-971.
101. Matthews KA, Haynes SG: The Type A behavior pattern and coronary risk: Update and critical evaluation. *Am J Epidem* 1986;123:923-960.

2

Psychologic Assessment in Cardiac Rehabilitation*

James A. Blumenthal

INTRODUCTION

Although the death rates from coronary heart disease (CHD) finally appear to be declining, heart disease still remains the most prevalent cause of death in this country. More than one million Americans suffer a myocardial infarction (MI) each year, and virtually every minute of every day someone is fatally stricken with an MI. For those fortunate enough to survive the event, the road to recovery can often be long and tedious.

As recently as 1970, a month or more of hospitalization was standard medical practice, and patients were often advised to have complete bed rest. After discharge, activity was discouraged, and sexual relations, travel, physical exercise, and return to work were often postponed for up to a year or, in some cases, for the remainder of the patient's life.

The rehabilitation of the cardiac patient has changed dramatically in the past 10 years. The limitations previously placed upon cardiac patients are presently considered too restrictive. Today it is not uncommon for patients with an uncomplicated MI to be discharged from the hospital in 7 to 10 days and to participate in supervised cardiac rehabilitation (CR) programs 6 to 8 weeks

---

*This work was supported in part by grants from the John D. and Catherine T. MacArthur Foundation and from the National Heart, Lung, and Blood Institute (RO1 30675-01A2).

after their infarctions. Many university teaching hospitals, as well as a growing number of community hospitals, local YMCAs, and privately funded fitness centers, now offer formal CR programs based on guidelines outlined by the American Heart Association[1] and the American College of Sports Medicine.[2]

Among the requirements for CR certification in several states is the regulation that every CR patient undergo a psychologic evaluation, as well as a medical evaluation, and that a variety of psychologic and behavioral treatment modalities be made available to those patients requiring assistance. The focus of the present chapter will be limited to issues of psychologic assessment for outpatients undergoing CR.

DEVELOPING A MULTIDIMENSIONAL CONCEPTUAL FRAMEWORK

A discussion of assessment procedures must begin with the basic question - assessment of what? To answer this question requires a broad-based conceptual framework in which the patient's condition is evaluated in a psychosocial context. I suggest a multidimensional assessment framework that permits assessment of the patient's ability to function in a variety of areas. This approach should not be confused with the multidisciplinary approach to CR, in which professionals from different disciplines - nursing, nutrition, medicine, exercise physiology, psychology - provide independent assessments of the patient with respect to their own special areas. A multidimensional framework, conducted by a single clinician, assumes that assessment of multiple life areas is important for (a) understanding how the patient is functioning in society and (b) guiding efforts to restore the patient to an optimal level of function.

The cardiac patient is not a psychiatric patient. Therefore, clinicians trained in the traditional "mental health" model may have to change their strategies and techniques. Many patients are not in acute distress and neither seek nor need traditional psychotherapy. Rather, the patient has experienced a significant change in health status and now suffers from a physical condition that affects, and is affected by, his or her ability to function psychologically, socially, and behaviorally.

The first and perhaps most difficult problem facing the clinician evaluating a cardiac patient is the problem of establishing rapport. Patients' pre-existing beliefs about psychology are often incongruent with their expectations regarding treatment for their medical condition. Some patients may express their concerns directly by saying that they resent the need for evaluation and that they are "not crazy"; others may indicate that they feel coerced by their physician or by the CR staff to be evaluated by a psychologist. The CR staff may also have misconceptions about the role of a psychologist, and thus may reinforce patients' notions that they are being referred because something is wrong with them. Indirect expressions of anger and resentment are not uncommon. For example, patients' resistance may take the form of noncompliance. There are several reasons for their reluctance to participate in psychologic assessment. The terms *psychology* and *psychiatry* may have negative connotations. For many patients, referral to a psychologist for evaluation suggests that their problems are "mental," which implies that they are not competent to cope with their condition. For patients who are already feeling helpless, assessment of their psychologic status can be extremely threatening. These patients often approach the psychologic evaluation as an opportunity to prove their mental health rather than as an opportunity to allow their doctor to know them better, to discuss their feelings, to learn more about their condition, or to develop better coping skills.

Several strategies are suggested for successfully avoiding the defensiveness and uncooperativeness that can accompany the initial visit. First, it is important that the psychologist be presented as part of the CR team. The relationship can be reinforced by the psychologist's participation at meetings where other CR staff are present (e.g., exercise sessions) and by having the psychologist located within a traditional medical facility, such as a hospital or medical clinic, rather than a mental health facility. Second, it is important that the psychologist clarify the reasons for the evaluation. For example, I reassure patients that their evaluation is routine (they are not being singled out because of some emotional problem) and emphasize that the goal of the assessment procedures is to evaluate "the whole person." Next, the psychologist should ask the patient to summarize in his or her own words what has happened to necessitate CR. In order to develop good rapport with cardiac patients, one must allow them to describe their physical condition in their own words. Most patients then begin to feel more comfortable, since they have been given an opportunity to talk about a subject of great importance to them and are able to demonstrate that they are knowledgeable about the topic. Next, the psychologist asks what the patients think may have caused their condition; this serves to assess patients' knowledge of risk factors and often provides an opportunity to educate them about CHD. It can be explained that a life-threatening illness frequently affects people's "mental attitude" - it is not uncommon for patients to experience a change in work, finances, family situation, mood, recreational activities, or sexual function.

At this point, the interview becomes less structured; however, I generally cover five interrelated areas of psychosocial function (for a more complete discussion, see Blumenthal[3]).

PERSONALITY FUNCTIONING AND PSYCHOPATHOLOGY

Emotional reactions always accompany MIs (see Tesar and Hackett, p. 67). Indeed, Cassem and Hackett[4] have used the term "ego infarction" to describe the psychologic impact of heart disease on the individual. In one study,[5] 80% of patients in the cardiac care unit (CCU) had some signs of anxiety, 58% were depressed, 22% were hostile, and 16% were agitated. Anxiety is usually the first emotional reaction to an MI. The content of anxious thought frequently focuses on fear of death, apprehension of further damage, concern with the significance of various somatic symptoms such as pain or dyspnea, and fear of being abandoned and isolated. Depression often follows and may persist for up to a year or longer. Many patients express fears of loss of income, sexual function, autonomy, and physical abilities. Anger is also not uncommon. Cardiac patients often feel frustrated by restrictions placed upon their activities and threatened by being placed in a dependent role in which they experience a lack of control. When assessing emotional reactions, it is also important to evaluate how patients cope with their feelings. Patients who claim that they were never afraid or insist that there is nothing wrong with them are practicing denial (the most common defense mechanism). In contrast with patients using denial, patients who use "isolation of affect" are aware of having had an MI but do not experience the natural feelings of anxiety or depression associated with the illness. Regression is seen less frequently, but is often a precursor of cardiac neurosis, a condition in which patients are extremely fearful about their physical integrity and adopt an overly passive and dependent sick role. These patients often become extremely debilitated; "secondary gain" (e.g., attention, sympathy, disability compensation, avoidance of adult responsibilities) may serve to perpetuate their maladaptive adjustment.

Successful coping has been shown to be associated with a better prognosis following MI. For example, several studies have shown that cardiac patients who failed to adequately adjust to their illness while in the CCU had higher mortalities in the first 6 months following discharge from the hospital than patients who were judged to be better adjusted[6-8] (see also chapters by Tesar and Hackett, p. 67 and Kinchla and Weiss, p. 133).

There are numerous instruments for measuring anxiety and depression. Self-rating forms are popular because they are brief, easily administered and scored, and relatively easy to interpret. The most common self-rating scales for depression are the Zung Self-Rating Depression Scale[9] and the Beck Depression Inventory.[10] Comparable self-report measures for assessing anxiety include the Taylor Manifest Anxiety Scale,[11] Spielberger State-Trait Anxiety Questionnaire,[12] and the Zung Self-Rating Anxiety Scale.[13] It should be noted, however, that these self-rating forms have a number of limitations. They are subject to distortion and response bias (e.g., denial), and they should not be relied on exclusively for diagnostic purposes. To some extent, the problem of response bias may be solved by including instruments that measure defensiveness and social desirability in conjunction with the self-rating scales. For example, the Edwards Social Desirability Scale[14] or the Marlowe-Crowne Social Desirability Scale[15] can be used in combination with the rating scales listed above. Other self-report inventories, such as the Profile of Mood States[16] or the Hopkins Symptom Checklist,[17] measure multiple affective states. Unfortunately, these measures also fail to assess the patient's test-taking attitude. Several self-report measures have been constructed to incorporate test-taking attitude. The best known multiple-scale inventory is the Minnesota Multiphasic Personality Inventory (MMPI).[18] The MMPI is a 566-item true/false questionnaire that yields four validity scales, 10 clinical scales, and a variety of experimental scales, including measures of anxiety, hostility, and ego strength. Comprehensive handbooks and numerous interpretative guides for MMPI results are available.[19,20]

Observer rating scales are another class of assessment instruments that may be particularly useful for evaluating psychopathology. For example, the Hamilton Psychiatric Rating Scale[21] and the Schedule for Affective Disorders and Schizophrenia[22] have been used for the diagnosis and estimation of the severity of symptoms of depression, and the Zung Anxiety Status Inventory[23] and the Hamilton Anxiety Scale[24] have been used to measure anxiety.

NEUROPSYCHOLOGIC FUNCTION

Screening for gross cognitive impairment is often appropriate in CR settings. Birren[25] has noted that "while age appears to be accompanied by normal psychophysiological slowing, it is exacerbated by the presence of disease, particularly those diseases of a stress character." For the patient who has undergone cardiac surgery, cognitive changes may be even more common. Memory loss, reduced concentration and attention, and, less frequently, aphasic signs (e.g., difficulty remembering a particular word, sensory loss, decreased fine motor control, or inability to perform simple arithmetic tasks) can be observed in some cardiac patients (Kinchla and Weiss, Chapter 9). Screening for cognitive dysfunction may alert the CR staff to important cognitive limitations that may have a bearing on the patient's medical management. For example, the patient with a hearing aid often finds a noisy gymnasium to be extremely aversive and may, as a result, be absent from exercise sessions without explanation; or the patient who is unable to comprehend or remember specific instructions may be noncompliant if a complex drug regimen is prescribed.

Although cognitive deficits can be assessed during a clinical interview, there are a number of standardized instruments that can aid the clinician in evaluating the presence and extent of cognitive impairment. The Mini-Mental State examination,[26] for example, consists of only 11 questions and requires less than 10 minutes to administer. The items measure orientation, attention, verbal recall, arithmetic skills, language function, and visual-motor integration.

The Russell Revised Wechsler Memory Scale[27] is a brief, easily administered test of memory function that yields objective scores of short- and long-term verbal (paragraph recall) and visual (reproduction of geometric designs) memory. Raw scores may be converted to a six-point scale for rating the severity of impairment. Another common screening instrument for general cognitive impairment is the Trail Making Test (TMT).[28] The TMT requires patients to connect, in sequence, a series of circles in numeric or alphabetic order.

A brief screening test for aphasias is the Halstead-Reitan Aphasia Screening Test[29] - an inexpensive, reliable, and rapidly administered instrument that assesses receptive and expressive language, simple arithmetic skills, and psychomotor function. A sensory perceptual examination is also available to evaluate the relative efficiency of the left and right sides of the body in recording auditory, visual, and tactile sensory input.

It should be emphasized that since normative data on older, medically ill patients is frequently unavailable, it may be difficult for many clinicians to determine the clinical significance of the test scores. However, standardized assessment can provide a baseline for future comparisons, and collection of data during an initial evaluation can provide an opportunity to measure change in cognitive function over the course of the patient's rehabilitation.

PHYSICAL HEALTH STATUS

The assessment of health status of the coronary patient is of primary concern for the psychologist and the physician. Review of cardiovascular risk factors, particularly those with a behavioral component - smoking, blood lipids, body weight, alcohol consumption, blood pressure, and Type A behavior - should have a high priority. There is also a broad range of health-related issues that are relevant to cardiac rehabilitation and that should be covered in the assessment.

SELF-PERCEIVED HEALTH STATUS

The cardiac patient's perception of his or her own health is important for several reasons. First, perceived health is closely correlated with general morale or life satisfaction. Second, perceived health is related to the likelihood of the patient's seeking further medical care. A simple four-point rating scale (excellent, good, fair, and poor) has been demonstrated to agree with physicians' ratings and to be better than physicians' ratings at predicting future patient ratings.[30] Third, self-ratings of health can be predictive of adjustment after illness. For example, health ratings have been found to predict morale after heart surgery,[31] return to work,[32] and, in our own program, adherence to exercise prescription.[33] Other more extensive self-report questionnaires can also be used, for example, the Cornell Medical Index,[34] a 195-item questionnaire based on a yes/no format. The Cornell Medical Index yields 12 physical symptom scales and six psychologic scales.

PAIN

Angina pectoris is often present in patients participating in CR. Seven pain dimensions should be covered: sensation, location, intensity, frequency, duration, precipitating factors, and relieving factors. A number of standard instruments can assist the clinician in obtaining these data. For example, the McGill Pain Questionnaire[35] can be used to assess verbal descriptions of pain. The McGill Pain Questionnaire is a 102-adjective checklist divided into 20 categories that describe three major dimensions of pain: sensory, affective, and evaluative. The McGill Pain Questionnaire yields measures of pain quality and intensity. Other measures of pain intensity include magnitude estimation and visual analogue scales. Magnitude estimation procedures involve asking patients to rate their pain numerically (e.g., on a scale from 0 to 10) or verbally (e.g., none, moderate, or severe). Visual analogue scales usually take the form of line segments (often 100 mm in length) with end points anchored by descriptive terms such as "no pain" and "worst pain ever felt." The patient is asked to draw a mark on the line indicating the level of pain experienced at the time. The visual analogue and the magnitude estimation procedures are strongly correlated with each other, although the visual analogue scale may be more sensitive to variations in pain intensity. Measures of pain location can be made using a pain map.[36] In this procedure, the patient is asked to indicate on the map where pain is experienced. Another method for pain assessment is the behavioral diary. Requesting that patients keep records about the frequency and duration of pain episodes and indicate precipitating factors (e.g., physical exertion or emotional stress) and relieving factors (e.g., rest or nitroglycerin) can provide the clinician with important information.

FUNCTIONAL CAPACITY

In CR settings, functional capacity is almost always assessed by exercise treadmill testing and quantified in MET (metabolic equivalent) units. It is estimated that 40% of all cardiac patients report that they are less active 6 months after their MIs. Although I am unaware of any activity survey designed specifically for cardiac patients, there are several activities of daily living questionnaires that may be useful for the more impaired patient. These instruments assess the degree and type of help required by the patient in coping with the daily demands of living. The greater the need for help, the greater the need for social resources. Behaviors focused on in assessment of activities of daily living include basic physical functions - such as eating, dressing, and grooming - and being able to shop, travel places outside of walking distance, cook meals, do housework, take appropriate medicine, and handle financial matters. Several standardized instruments are available, including the OARS MFAQ,[37] the Katz's Index of Independence and Activities of Daily Living,[38] and the Instrumental Activities of Daily Living scale.[39]

MEDICATION

Most patients participating in CR programs are required to take medication. Psychologists should always be aware of the kind of medications a patient is taking and the ability of the patient to adhere to the pharmacologic regimen. An excellent discussion of the problems of noncompliance with prescribed medications is presented by Epstein and Cluss.[40]

HEALTH CARE UTILIZATION

It is important for the psychologist to be aware of the patient's pattern of health care utilization. Once a person has experienced an MI, good health can no longer be taken for granted. Many patients become sensitized to their physical health; in extreme cases, they may become preoccupied with it and over-react to any physical sensations. The person who is overly concerned about his or her condition may engage in a variety of maladaptive behaviors, including "doctor shopping," frequent trips to the emergency room, and solicitation of information and advice from different members of the CR team. These patients are often troublesome for CR staff, because they tend to be demanding and never seem to receive the reassurance they need. Their behavior is often self-defeating: patients may get conflicting messages that serve to heighten their anxiety, or they may alienate the CR staff and thus frustrate their dependency needs. The other extreme behavioral style is that of the "deniers" who avoid medical contact and do not advise the CR team of symptoms or changes in health status. By failing to communicate information to the CR staff, these patients are at greater risk for fatal and nonfatal CHD events.

STRESS AND TYPE A BEHAVIOR PATTERN

Most patients believe that stress contributed to their illness, and empirical research generally supports this belief.[41] For example, studies have shown that an accumulation of life changes (e.g., death of a loved one, divorce, or unemployment) occurs in the year preceding the clinical manifestations of CHD.[42] There are a number of self-report measures of life change, including the Social Readjustment Rating Scale, the Schedule of Recent Events,[43] and the Life Experience Survey.[44] The last scale is more flexible than the others, in that it allows the patient to rate the degree (on a one to five scale) and impact (positive or negative) of the life event.

The Type A behavior pattern is now established as a risk factor for CHD. Type A individuals are approximately twice as likely to develop CHD as their Type B counterparts, and are also more prone to recurrent infarctions and progression of coronary atherosclerosis.[45] Type A individuals are hard-driving, competitive, aggressive, and impatient. Type B individuals, on the other hand, are more relaxed and easy-going (Thoresen et al., Chapter 7). Classification of individuals as Type A or B is usually determined by a clinical judgment based on a series of specific questions during a structured interview.[46] The questions are designed to elicit a particular type of response that is often displayed by Type A individuals, as well as to acquire information regarding the individual's typical behavior based on self-reported attitudes and practices. During the structured interview, the subject is asked approximately 20 to 25 questions dealing with feelings of ambition and competitiveness, past history of feelings of anger, sense of time urgency and impatience, and current feelings of irritation and frustration. The interview is conducted in a manner designed to create a situation that will actually elicit Type A characteristics. For example, the interviewer purposely interrupts the subject to elicit anger, asks questions rapidly to encourage a quick response, and purposely stammers over several questions to provoke an interruption. Expressive speech style, particularly loud and rapid speech, frequent interruptions, and the potential for hostility appear to be most strongly correlated with structured interview ratings.[47] Thus, such assessment of the Type A behavior pattern depends more on observed overt behaviors than on the patient's self-reported practices.

Although the interview method is widely recognized as the most valid measure of Type A behavior, it requires training for administration and classification, and it has been criticized for being too global and subjective. As a result, psychologists have attempted to develop more objective paper-and-pencil questionnaires to assess Type A characteristics.

The Jenkins Activity Survey for Health Prediction (JAS) is the most widely used self-report measure of Type A behavior.[48] The JAS yields an overall Type A score and three-factor analytically derived subscales: "speed and impatience," "job involvement," and "hard-driving and competitive." The development and validation of the JAS has been reported in detail elsewhere.[49,50] Scores on the Type A scale of the JAS have been shown to be both prospectively and retrospectively correlated with increased risk of primary and secondary CHD events, although its predictive value for MI appears to be weaker than that of the structured interview.[45] However, the JAS also suffers from a number of shortcomings: it is relatively expensive to administer and score by computer, it requires up to 25 minutes to score by hand, and the Type A scale has a relatively low correlation with the structured interview and with CHD risk. As a result, too many patients may be misclassified by the JAS, if the structured interview is considered the standard. Other self-report measures have been developed, including our own Type A Self-Rating Inventory.[51] However, the clinical efficacy of the scales has not been demonstrated.

SOCIAL AND WORK ADJUSTMENT

SOCIAL SUPPORT

Social support may be defined as the availability of people on whom the patient can rely, people who make the patient feel valued, loved, and cared about. Although there are numerous ways in which social support may be defined, most definitions indicate that social support involves the perception that there is a sufficient number of available others to whom one can turn in times of need and a degree of satisfaction with the available support. A number of studies reviewed by Cobb[52] and Dean and Lin[53] indicate that good social support buffers the effects of stress on illness. For example, Berkman and Syme[54] found that people who lack social and community ties were more than twice as likely to die in a 9-year follow-up study than those with more extensive contacts, and Gore[55] showed that among individuals faced with the stress of unemployment, those with little social support have significantly higher elevations and more changes in measures of serum cholesterol level, illness symptoms, and affective response than the group with more social support. In addition, two studies[56,57] suggested that psychologic intervention (e.g., group therapy) can facilitate early return to work, reduce emotional disturbance, and minimize post-MI complications, although differences in mortalities between treatment and control groups were not statistically significant.

Among the measures of social support presently available, the Social Support Questionnaire[58] is one of the more promising methods for quantifying social support. It is a 27-item questionnaire that requires respondents to list the people on whom they can rely in a given situation and to indicate how satisfied they are with these social supports.

MARRIAGE

Heart disease affects the spouse as well as the patient, and it has been suggested that while the patient may recover, the spouse may not.[59] Spouses of patients often display anxiety and depression, but are seldom included in CR treatment. Therefore, the spouse should almost always be included in the assessment procedure. Several self-report measures of global marital satisfaction can be used to assess marital adjustment.[60,61]

Conflicts over compliance with prescribed medical treatment are common, even in "healthy" marriages. For example, it has been reported that 6 to 9 months after an MI, emotional problems are present in three-quarters of all families studied as a result of "differences over medical instructions."[62] Therefore, it is important that patient and spouse be clear as to what the instructions are, and aware of what behaviors are and are not permitted. More quarrels could be avoided if the patient and spouse knew whether the patient's raking leaves or doing light housework was considered safe.

Another common problem for the post-MI patient and spouse is the successful return to the prior level of sexual activity. It has been documented that the level of sexual activity reported by persons 1 year after an MI is about 60% of activity prior to illness, and less than half of the post-MI patients resume the same frequency of sexual intercourse as before the infarct.[63] Patients attribute their decreased sexual activity to a variety of reasons, including loss of interest, spousal reluctance, depression, and anxiety. Unfortunately, patients and physicians tend to be uncomfortable when discussing sexual matters openly; as a result, this area tends to be ignored. All too often, advice on sexual activity either is not given or is presented in terms so global (e.g., "just take it easy") that it is useless to most patients. Masters and Johnson[64] reported that up to two-thirds of patients who suffer MIs do not receive any advice from the medical team about sexual functioning, and it has been shown that less information is given to cardiac patients about sexual activity than about other activities, such as work, physical exertion, or diet. Curiously, data suggest that while physicians report that they do counsel their patients about sexuality, most patients report that they receive no such counseling. Most patients would like to know more about how their condition affects their sexual activity; an excellent text is available[65] for such information.

WORK

Most evidence suggests that the majority of patients who have suffered an MI return to work within the first year after the event.[66] Approximately 50% return to work at the end of 3 months, 80% by 6 months, and 90% at the end of 1 year. A number of psychologic and demographic variables predict whether or not an individual will return to work, including age, severity of cardiac damage, socioeconomic status, and level of psychologic impairment. In addition, the patient who enjoys work is more likely to be motivated to return to work, particularly if the physical demands of the job do not exceed the patient's limitations.

The five psychosocial domains reviewed above reflect a comprehensive assessment of the patient and his or her environment. This assessment must be combined with the assessments made by other members of the CR team so that a coordinated treatment program can be developed. Those readers interested in the psychologic treatment aspects of CR are referred elsewhere,[67,68] as well as to the other chapters in this book.

CONCLUSION

Coronary heart disease (CHD) is a condition with significant psychologic and social, as well as physical, consequences. As such, psychologic assessment is an important component of any cardiac rehabilitation (CR) program. A multidimensional framework is proposed, with particular emphasis on five psychosocial domains: personality function and psychopathology, neuropsychologic function, physical health status, stress and Type A behavior, and social and work adjustment. The results of the psychologic assessment should emphasize the relative strengths and adaptive resources of the patient, as well as problem areas. Efforts should also be made to integrate psychologic test results with evaluations from other disciplines within the CR team so that a coordinated treatment program can be formulated (see Chapter 10).

REFERENCES

1. *The Exercise Standards Book.* Dallas, American Heart Association, 1979.
2. American College of Sports Medicine: *Guidelines for Graded Exercise Testing and Exercise Prescription.* 2nd Ed. Philadelphia, Lea & Febiger, 1980.
3. Blumenthal JA: Assessment of patients with coronary heart disease, in Keefe FJ, Blumenthal JA (eds): *Assess-*

ment *Strategies in Behavioral Medicine.* New York, Grune & Stratton, 1982:37-97.
4. Cassem NH, Hackett TP: Psychological rehabilitation of myocardial infarction patients in the acute phase. *Heart Lung* 1973;2:382-388.
5. Hackett TP, Cassem NH, Wishnie HA: The coronary care unit: An appraisal of its psychological hazards. *N Engl J Med* 1968;279:1365-1370.
6. Cromwell R: *Stress, Personality and Nursing Care in Myocardial Infarction.* Washington, DC, National Institutes of Mental Health, Grants MH-09220 and MH-13614, 1969.
7. Garrity TF, Klein RF: A behavioral prediction of survival among heart attack patients, in Palmer E, Jeffers FC (eds): *Predictions of Life Span.* Lexington, MA, Health Publishing Co, 1971:215-222.
8. Gentry WD, Foster S, Haney T: Denial as a determinant of anxiety and perceived health status in the coronary care unit. *Psychosom Med* 1972;34:39-44.
9. Zung WWK: A self-rating depression scale. *Arch Gen Psychiatry* 1965;12:63-70.
10. Beck AT, Ward CH, Mendelson M, Mock JE, Erbaugh J: An inventory for measuring depression. *Arch Gen Psychiatry* 1961;4:561-571.
11. Taylor J: A personality scale of manifest anxiety. *J Abnorm Soc Psychol* 1955;48:285-290.
12. Spielberger CE, Gorsuch RL, Luschene RE: *Manual for the State-Trait Anxiety Inventory.* Palo Alto, CA, Consulting Psychologist Press, 1970.
13. Zung WWK: A rating instrument for anxiety disorders. *Psychosomatics* 1971;12:371-379.
14. Edwards AL: *Edwards Personal Preference Schedule.* New York, The Psychological Corporation, 1953.
15. Crowne DP, Marlowe D: *The Approval Motive.* New York, John Wiley & Sons, 1967.
16. McNair DM, Lorr M, Droppleman LF: *Profile of Mood States: Manual.* San Diego, CA, Educational and Industrial Testing Service, 1971.
17. Derogatis L, Lipman RS, Rickels K, Uhlenhuth EH, Covi L: The Hopkins symptom checklist (HSCL): A measure of primary symptom dimensions, in Pichot P (ed): *Psychological Measurements in Psychopharmacology: Modern Problems in Pharmacopsychiatry,* vol. 7. Basel, S. Karger, 1974.
18. Hathaway SR, McKinley JC: *The Minnesota Multiphasic Personality Inventory Manual.* Minneapolis, University of Minnesota Press, 1943.

19. Carson RC: Interpretive manual to the MMPI, in Butcher JN (ed): *MMPI: Research Developments and Clinical Applications.* New York, McGraw-Hill, 1969:279-296.
20. Lacher D: *The MMPI: Clinical Assessment and Automated Interpretation.* Los Angeles, Western Psychological Services, 1974.
21. Hamilton M: Development of a rating scale for primary depressive illness. *Br J Soc Clin Psychol* 1967;6:278-296.
22. Spitzer RL, Endicott J: *Schedule for Affective Disorders and Schizophrenia - Life-Times Version (SADS-L).* New York, New York Psychiatric Institute, 1977.
23. Zung, WWK: The depression status inventory: An adjunct to the self-rating depression scale. *J Clin Psychol* 1972;28:539-543.
24. Hamilton M: Development of a rating scale for primary depressive illness. *Br J Soc Clin Psychol* 1967;6:278-296.
25. Birren JE: Translations in gerontology from lab to life: Physiology and speed of response. *Am Psychol* 1974;29:808-815.
26. Folstein MF, Folstein SE, McHugh PE: Mini-mental state. A practical method for grading the cognitive state of patients for the clinician. *J Psychiatr Res* 1975;12:189-198.
27. Russell EW: The multiple scoring method for the assessment of complex memory functions. *J Consult Clin Psychol* 1975;43:800-809.
28. Reitan RM: Validity of the Trail Making Test as an indicator of organic brain damage. *Percept Mot Skills* 1958;8:271-276.
29. Heimberger RF, Reitan RM: Easily administered written test for lateralizing brain lesions. *J Neurosurg* 1961;181:301-312.
30. Maddox GL, Douglass EB: Self-assessment of health: A longitudinal study of elderly subjects. *J Health Soc Behav* 1973;14:87-93.
31. Brown JS, Rawlinson M: The morale of patients following open heart surgery. *J Health Soc Behav* 1976;17:139-144.
32. Garrity TF: Vocational adjustment after first myocardial infarction: Comparative assessment of several variables suggested in the literature. *Soc Sci Med* 1973;7:705-707.
33. Blumenthal JA, Williams RS, Wallace AG, Williams RB, Needels T: Physiological and psychological variables

predict adherence to prescribed medical therapy in patients recovering from myocardial infarction. *Psychosom Med* 1982;44:519-527.
34. Brodman K, Erdmann AJ, Lorge I, Wolff NG: The Cornell Medical Index: An adjunct to medical interview. *JAMA* 1949;140:530-534.
35. Melzack R: The McGill pain questionnaire: Major properties and scoring methods. *Pain* 1975;1:277-299.
36. Keele KD: The pain chart. *Lancet* 1948;2:6-8.
37. OARS: *Multidimensional Functional Assessment: The OARS Methodology: A Manual.* 2nd Ed. Durham, NC, Center for the Study of Aging and Human Development, 1978.
38. Katz S, Ford AB, Moskowitz RW, Jackson BA, Jaffe MW: Studies of illness in the aged: The index of ADL, a standardized measure of biological and psychosocial function. *JAMA* 1963;185:914-919.
39. Lawton MP, Brody E: Assessment of older people: Self-maintaining and instrumental activities of daily living. *Gerontologist* 1969;9:179-186.
40. Epstein LH, Cluss PA: A behavioral medicine perspective on adherence to long-term medical regimens. *J Consult Clin Psychol* 1982;50:950-971.
41. Jenkins CD: Recent evidence supporting psychological and social risk factors for coronary disease. *N Engl J Med* 1976;294:987-994, 1033-1038.
42. Theorell T: Life events before and after the onset of a premature myocardial infarction, in Gunderson EKE, Rahe RH (eds): *Stressful Life Events: Their Nature and Effects.* Springfield, IL, Charles C. Thomas, 1974:101-117.
43. Holmes TH, Rahe RH: The social readjustment rating scale. *J Psychosom Res* 1967;11:219-225.
44. Sarason IG, Johnson JH, Siegel JM: Assessing the impact of life changes: Development of the life experiences survey. *J Consult Clin Psychol* 1978;46:932-946.
45. The Review Panel on Coronary Prone Behavior and Coronary Heart Disease: Coronary-prone behavior and coronary heart disease: A critical review. *Circulation* 1981;63:1199-1215.
46. Rosenman RH: The interview method of assessment of the coronary prone behavior pattern, in Dembroski TM, Weiss SM, Shields JL, Haynes SG, Feinlab M (eds): *Coronary Prone Behavior.* New York, Springer-Verlag, 1978:55-69.

47. Blumenthal JA, O'Toole L, Haney T: Behavioral assessment of the type A behavior pattern. *Psychosom Med* 1984;46:415-423.
48. Jenkins CD, Rosenman RH, Friedman M: Development of an objective psychological test for the determination of the coronary prone behavior pattern in employed men. *J Chronic Dis* 1967;20:371-379.
49. Jenkins CD, Zyzanski SH, Rosenman RH: Progress toward validation of a computer-scored test for the type A coronary prone behavior pattern. *Psychosom Med* 1971; 33:193-201.
50. Zyzanski SJ, Jenkins SD: Basic dimensions within the coronary prone behavior pattern. *J Chronic Dis* 1970;22:781-795.
51. Blumenthal JA, Herman S, O'Toole L, Haney TL, Williams RB, Barefoot, JC: Development of a brief self-report measure of the Type A (coronary prone) behavior pattern. *J Psychosom Res* 1985;29:265-274.
52. Cobb S: Social support as a moderator of life stress. *Psychosom Med* 1976;38:300-314.
53. Dean A, Lin N: The stress-buffering role of social support. *J Nerv Ment Dis* 1977;165:403-417.
54. Berkman LF, Syme SC: Social networks, host resistance, and mortality: A nine-year follow-up study of Alameda County residents. *Am J Epidemiol* 1979;109:186-204.
55. Gore S: The effect of social support in moderating the health consequences of coemployment. *J Health Soc Behav* 1978;19:157-165.
56. Ibrahim MA, Feldman JG, Sultz HA, Staiman MG, Young LJ, Dean D: Management after myocardial infarction: A controlled trial of the effect of group psychotherapy. *Psychiatry Med* 1974;5:253-268.
57. Rahe RH, Ward HW, Hayes V: Brief group therapy in myocardial infarction rehabilitation: Three to four-year follow-up of a controlled trial. *Psychosom Med* 1979;41:229-242.
58. Sarason IG, Levine HM, Basham RB, Sarason BR: Assessing social support: The social support questionnaire. *J Pers Soc Psychol* 1983;44:127-139.
59. Crawshaw JE: Community rehabilitation after acute myocardial infarction. *Heart Lung* 1974;3:258-271.
60. Spanier GB: Measuring dyadic adjustment: New scales for assessing the quality of marriage and similar dyads. *Journal of Marriage and Family* 1976;38:15-28.
61. Schutz W: *MATE, A Firo Awareness Scale* (revised). Palo Alto, CA, Consulting Psychologists Press, 1976.

62. Wishnie HA, Hackett TP, Cassem NH: Psychological hazards of convalescence following myocardial infarction, *JAMA* 1971;215:1291-1296.
63. Hellerstein HK, Friedman EH: Sexual activity and the post coronary patient. *Arch Intern Med* 1970;125:987-999.
64. Masters WH, Johnson VE: *Human Sexual Response.* Boston, Little, Brown & Co, 1966.
65. Scheingold LD, Wagner NN: *Sound Sex and the Aging Heart.* New York, Human Science Press, 1974.
66. Williams RB, Gentry WD: Psychological problems inherent in the cardiopathic state, in Long C (ed): *Prevention and Rehabilitation in Ischemic Heart Disease.* Baltimore, Williams & Wilkins, 1980:106-128.
67. Doehrman SR: Psychological aspects of recovery from coronary heart disease: A review. *Soc Sci Med* 1977;11:199-218.
68. Blanchard EB, Miller ST: Psychological treatment of cardiovascular disease. *Arch Gen Psychiatr* 1977;34:1402-1413.

3

Coping with the Sequelae of Smoking Cessation*

Neil E. Grunberg and Deborah J. Bowen

INTRODUCTION

Cigarette smoking is the single most preventable cause of premature death and illness in the United States. Roughly one-third of all cardiovascular problems are associated with cigarette smoking and 170,000 annual deaths from coronary heart disease (CHD) are directly related to cigarette smoking. Myocardial infarction (MI), sudden cardiac death, arteriosclerotic aneurysm of the aorta, arteriosclerotic peripheral vascular disease, and other cardiovascular diseases may result from habitual cigarette smoking.[1,2] These facts should come as no surprise, and there is little need to preach to readers of this book about the importance of smoking cessation and maintenance of cessation by cardiac patients. Instead, our intention is to discuss the sequelae of smoking cessation and how to cope with these effects. Emphasis is placed on information that may be used to help the cardiac patient deal with the consequences of smoking cessation in order to maintain abstinence.

---

*The opinions or assertions contained herein are the private ones of the authors and are not to be construed as official or reflecting the views of the USUHS or the Department of Defense.

CESSATION OF CIGARETTE SMOKING

OVERVIEW

The majority of habitual smokers who quit smoking do so on their own.[3] However, less than 25% of smokers who give it up continue to abstain 1 year after quitting.[4] There are, however, notable exceptions to these bleak statistics. In particular, individuals who believe that they are at personal risk if they keep smoking (such as cardiac patients) are more likely to quit and remain abstinent. One study reported that roughly 50% of smokers with CHD (i.e., MI or angina) quit smoking and maintained abstinence more than 4 years later.[5] When individuals receive intensive advice from health-care professionals to quit smoking, they are more likely to quit and remain abstinent.[6,7] For example, 62% of patients with MI who were strongly advised to quit smoking by their physicians and nurses were still abstinent a few years later.[8] However, while encouraging, these statistics reflect the fact that many high-risk patients return to this life-threatening habit. For this reason, it is important to be familiar with smoking cessation programs and techniques and ways to help patients cope with the sequelae of smoking cessation that may lead to relapse.

CESSATION TECHNIQUES

There are a variety of smoking cessation programs and approaches that may help those patients who do not quit on their own. A list of local programs appears in the Yellow Pages of most telephone directories under "Smokers' Information and Treatment Centers." These programs may be found in local hospitals, government health departments, community centers, universities, and medical centers. In addition, smoking cessation programs are sponsored by the American Heart Association, American Cancer Society, American Lung Association, and individual church groups (e.g., Five Day Plan of the Seventh Day Adventists). Programs range in price from nominal fees to hundreds of dollars. Some of these programs use self-help approaches, whereas other require several weeks of regular participation in a scheduled group. These programs include information about the harmful effects of smoking, behavioral self-control strategies (e.g., identifying and avoiding situations in which smoking is likely, substituting activities such as exercise), cognitive self-control strategies (e.g., mentally rehearsing reasons for not smoking), social support (e.g., encouragement from friends and family), hypnotherapy, drug treatments (e.g., nicotine chewing gum), and aversion strategies (e.g., rapid smoking). (See Pechacek[7] for a more detailed discussion of each of these programs and techniques.)

Individual patients will respond to different programs and approaches. It is important to help patients find those programs that suit their particular needs and individual preferences. The most effective treatments use several of these strategies. For cardiac patients, aversion strategies may be quite dangerous and probably should be avoided.[9] In addition, nicotine chewing gum (which may be a fine approach to help smokers who are at risk for cancer and chronic obstructive lung disease) may pose potential risks for cardiac patients because of the vasoconstrictive effects of nicotine.[10] Also, there are some suggestive data implicating nicotine as a cause of cardiac muscle abnormalities.[11]

HELPING SMOKERS ABSTAIN

There are a number of actions that health professionals can take in addition to referring patients to smoking cessation programs and advising them about therapeutic approaches. There is empirical evidence indicating that, in general, patients are particularly sensitive to direct advice from physicians and other health professionals to quit smoking.[12,13] Face-to-face intervention with follow-up is the most effective way to get people to quit smoking.[7] Furthermore, patients who are told by their physicians to quit and who are given literature about withdrawal symptoms and ways to cope with these symptoms have higher abstinence rates than do smokers who are told only to quit.[13] Unfortunately, surveys reveal that the minority of patients who smoke are advised by their physicians to quit.[14]

It is important that health professionals not smoke or that patients do not see them smoke. Modeling greatly affects cigarette smoking behavior.[15] Medical personnel also should provide information about the risks of smoking, convince patients that they can quit smoking, and reinforce maintenance of smoking cessation. Useful literature and materials for health professionals and patients may be obtained from the Office on Smoking and Health (Rockville, MD), Centers for Disease Control (Atlanta, GA), National Heart, Lung, and Blood Institute (Bethesda, MD), National Cancer Institute (Bethesda, MD), and the American Lung Association (New York City or local chapters). (See Lichtenstein and Danaher[6] for a detailed discussion of specific actions that medical personnel can take to encourage smoking cessation.) Moreover, patients should be prepared for the sequelae of smoking cessation and ways to cope with these effects.

SEQUELAE OF SMOKING CESSATION

Many smokers can successfully quit smoking, but the majority return to their habit. As Mark Twain wrote: "To cease smoking is the easiest thing I ever did; I ought to know because I've done it a thousand times."[16] Because cardiac patients are highly motivated to stop smoking, most probably will succeed. However, many of them will relapse within a year or less. Knowledge of the effects of smoking cessation and ways to deal with them help maintain abstinence.

The most common consequence of smoking cessation, besides relapse per se, is craving for cigarettes.[17] This is frequently situation-specific (e.g., at parties, during periods of stress) or associated with particular behaviors (e.g., drinking alcohol or coffee, talking on the phone).

Smokers who quit smoking also report or demonstrate signs of irritability, emotionality, anxiety, irascibility, and inability to concentrate.[17-21] Behavioral effects of smoking cessation include worsened performance on psychomotor tests (i.e., vigilance and tracking) and on difficult verbal memory tests.[18,22] Physical and biologic effects of smoking cessation include nausea, sleep disturbances, headache, gastrointestinal problems (e.g., cramps, constipation), and gains in body weight.[17,23-26] All of these effects may lead to a relapse. Other physiologic consequences of cessation that may contribute to relapse include changes in electroencephalographic activity, changes in metabolic activity (e.g., as measured by 30-minute post-prandial blood glucose and oxygen consumption), decreases in heart rate and diastolic blood pressure, and changes in urinary levels of norepinephrine and epinephrine.[27-29] It may be useful to inform patients of these effects so that they will prepare for them and will correctly attribute these consequences to smoking cessation. Failure to recognize components of the tobacco abstinence syndrome may lead to increased anxiety and fear in patients who think that they are generally "falling apart" mentally or physically. It is important to emphasize that the unpleasant effects of smoking cessation will eventually abate and disappear.

COPING WITH SEQUELAE OF SMOKING CESSATION

AVOIDING RELAPSE

As previously mentioned, a high percentage of even the most motivated ex-smokers will relapse within a year of cessation. It is important to emphasize to a patient that this commonly cited fact simply reflects the likelihood of success of one attempt to quit smoking.[30] Patients who smoke should be encouraged to keep trying to kick their habit because most people will succeed after repeated attempts. Encouragement is vital to help maintain their motivation and their belief that they can give up cigarettes for good.[6] In addition, it has been demonstrated that follow-up communication from health professionals to insure maintenance of smoking cessation (e.g., in person, by telephone, or by mail) increases the likelihood of long-term abstinence.[14]

Frequently, the craving for cigarettes will be most intense and difficult to resist in specific situations. To help patients cope with the temptation to smoke, it is useful to have them identify, list, and carry the list of situations in which they are at high risk for relapse. Awareness of the situations and stimuli that are associated with smoking usually helps the ex-smoker avoid relapse. Three common categories associated with high relapse rates are negative emotional states, interpersonal conflict, and social pressure.[31]

SELF-CONTROL STRATEGIES

In addition to identifying high-risk relapse situations and stimuli, behavioral and cognitive self-control strategies can be tailored to help patients resist the temptation to smoke.[32] For instance, if smoking was associated with morning coffee-drinking, it might be helpful to switch to a different drink. If smoking was likely in social situations, it might be helpful to rehearse and role-play refusal of offered cigarettes, or to substitute cigarettes with gum or mints. One cognitive self-control strategy is to think about harmful effects of smoking whenever craving becomes unbearable. Patients also might find it useful to remind themselves that they, and not the cigarettes, are in control. In general, substitution of behaviors (e.g., exercise) and thoughts (e.g., "I am an ex-smoker") for smoking are effective techniques to avoid relapse.[31,33] Patients should write and carry a list of specific coping strategies for those situations in which the risk of relapse is high.

Both behavioral and cognitive self-control strategies should be used to cope with craving and with other effects of smoking cessation.[34] For example, ex-smokers who experience irritability or anger with fellow workers, friends, or spouses should remind themselves that these reactions probably are related to withdrawal from cigarettes and should be dealt with accordingly: (a) behaviorally (e.g., walk away) and (b) cognitively (e.g., think about health benefits of quitting). Attributing any unpleasant psychologic and physical reactions that occur to withdrawal from cigarettes also tends to help people better cope with their responses and may help to avoid relapse.

SOCIAL SUPPORT

Another way to combat the adverse effects of smoking cessation is to enlist social support from spouses, friends, and co-workers.[35] The act of telling other people that one is about to quit smoking may, itself, help establish a commitment to succeed.[6] This social network can help the ex-smoker maintain abstinence by positively reinforcing smoking cessation and by understanding any bouts of irritability, anxiety, and so on by the ex-smoker. The person who is trying to quit should not be obsessively monitored.[35]

RELAXATION TRAINING

Relaxation techniques may be used to cope with situations in which relapse is likely and to deal with the stressful sequelae of smoking cessation. One approach is to first identify tension-producing situations. Then, one applies a pre-determined sequence of procedures (e.g., counting to 40, breathing deeply 10 times, or imagining a tranquil scene) while relaxing muscles starting from one extremity (e.g., feet) and proceeding throughout the body.[36] This type of approach has been used successfully to reduce various types of stress.[32,37] See Benson,[38] Davis and colleagues,[39] and McKay and associates,[40] for detailed descriptions of relaxation techniques.

CONTROLLING WEIGHT GAIN

One reason many people give for returning to smoking or refusing to quit in the first place is a concern about gaining weight.[41] It is true that many people who quit smoking do gain weight and that smokers generally weigh less than comparably aged nonsmokers.[24,26] Therefore, it is important to prepare patients for the possibility of weight gain and to deal with the weight gain as a specific problem in conjunction with smoking cessation. There are a variety of ways to control body weight, including diets, drugs, exercise, behavioral treatment, psychotherapy, hypnosis, surgery (in extreme cases of obesity), and a host of additional psychologic techniques (e.g., cognitive restructuring, relaxation therapy).

As with smoking cessation, the most effective techniques for weight loss depend on the individual patient. However, some generalizations can be made. Diets and fasting will result in weight loss, but people tend to discontinue their diets and regain the lost weight. Drug therapy may be useful but may have negative side effects - the agents used are not entirely safe. For example, some drugs (e.g., amphetamines) help reduce weight for a few weeks, but effectiveness decreases with usage and deleterious side effects appear (e.g., irritability, insomnia, possible drug abuse). Surgery (i.e., jejunoileal or gastric bypass) is effective, but it should only be used in the most extreme and recalcitrant cases of obesity because there are serious side effects associated with the procedures, including liver failure, renal failure, and possible death. In contrast, behavioral treatment may decrease body weight with few or no adverse side effects. Behavioral self-control techniques of food consumption in conjunction with exercise is a safe and effective approach to control body weight provided that the changes in lifestyle are maintained. Other psychologic techniques used to control body weight have received less empirical evaluation and therefore remain largely untested. Grunberg,[42] Powers,[43] and Stuart and co-workers[44] give detailed discussions and evaluations of weight control techniques. Patients may apply these techniques on their own or they can participate in a weight control program. Such programs are listed in local telephone directories under "Reducing and Weight Control Services" and may be found at hospitals, health departments, and community and medical centers.

Some recent research suggests ways to control body weight that may be particularly appropriate after cessation of smoking. Laboratory studies of animals indicate that body weight gains after cessation of nicotine intake (a primary pharmacologic agent in tobacco) result from the increased consumption of sweet-tasting foods and decreased physical activity.[24,45,46] Similarly, cigarette smoking in humans is inversely related to consumption of sweet-tasting foods.[24,47] These findings suggest that avoiding sweet-tasting foods and increasing exercise may be especially effective weight control techniques after cessation of smoking.

CONCLUSION

Maintenance of abstinence from cigarettes is difficult, but fortunately, most cardiac patients are highly motivated to give up cigarettes. Reminders of the health hazards of smoking, encouragement to quit, and positive reinforcement of cessation are particularly effective when communicated by health-care personnel. In addition, it may be useful to hand out relevant literature and to refer patients to smoking cessation programs and techniques. For patients who relapse, physicians should emphasize that repeated attempts will eventually succeed and the patient should keep trying to quit. Also, patients should be prepared for the physical and psychologic withdrawal symptoms of smoking cessation and should be provided with various coping techniques. Additional assistance could include smoking cessation follow-ups in routine office visits and a call-in service for ex-smokers who need to talk to someone when they are tempted to smoke or are suffering from withdrawal.

It does no good to paint an overly optimistic picture and thereby lose credibility with patients who suffer unpleasant withdrawal symptoms. However, that is not to will discourage anyone from trying to quit smoking. Instead, health professionals should emphasize the importance of abstinence and should help patients cope with the consequences of smoking cessation by identifying them as such and by suggesting ways to deal with these effects. The more active the role taken by health-care professionals, the greater the likelihood of successful abstinence by patients.

REFERENCES

1. *Smoking and Health: A Report of the Surgeon General*, publication 79-50066. US Department of Health, Education, and Welfare, Public Health Service, 1979.
2. *The Health Consequences of Smoking: Cardiovascular Disease*, publication 84-50204. US Department of Health and Human Services, Public Health Service, 1983.
3. Horn D: Who is quitting and why, in Schwartz, JL (ed): *Progress in Smoking Cessation: International Conference on Smoking Cessation*. New York, American Cancer Society, 1978:27-31.
4. Hunt WA, Matarazzo JD: Three years later: Recent developments in the experimental modification of smoking behavior. *J Abnorm Psychol* 1973;81:107-114.
5. Weinblatt E, Shapiro S, Frank CW: Changes in personal characteristics of men, over five years, following first diagnosis of coronary heart disease. *Am J Public Health* 1971;61:831-842.
6. Lichtenstein E, Danaher BG: What can the physician do to assist the patient to stop smoking, in Brashear RE, Rhodes ML (eds): *Chronic Obstructive Lung Disease*. St. Louis, CV Mosby, 1978:227-241.
7. Pechacek TF: Modification of smoking behavior, in Krasnegor, NA (ed): *The Behavioral Aspects of Smoking* (NIDA Research Monograph 26). Rockville, MD, Department of Health, Education, and Welfare, 1979:127-188.
8. Burt A, Thornley P, Illingworth D, White P, Shaw TRD, Turner R: Stopping smoking after myocardial infarction. *Lancet* 1974;1:304-306.
9. Lichtenstein E, Glasgow RE: Rapid smoking: Side effects and safeguards. *J Consult Clin Psychol* 1977;45:815-821.
10. Taylor P: Ganglionic stimulating and blocking agents, in Gilman AG, Goodman LS, Gilman A (eds): *The Pharma-*

cological Basis of Therapeutics. New York, Macmillan, 1980:211-219.
11. Morse DE: *Endocrinological Responses to the Administration of Nicotine: Interactions with Drug Initiation, Conditioned Effects, and Conditions of Stress* (thesis). Uniformed Services University of the Health Sciences, Bethesda, MD, 1984.
12. Raw M: Persuading people to stop smoking. *Behav Res Ther* 1976;14:97-101.
13. Russell MAH, Wilson C, Taylor C, Baker CD: Effect of general practitioners' advice against smoking. *Br Med J* 1979;28:231-235.
14. *Adult Use of Tobacco - 1975.* US Department of Health, Education, and Welfare, Public Health Service, 1976.
15. Pomerleau OF: Behavioral factors in the establishment, maintenance, and cessation of smoking, in *Smoking and Health: A Report of the Surgeon General,* publication 79-50066. US Department of Health, Education, and Welfare, Public Health Service, 1979.
16. Twain M, in Adams AK (ed): *The Home Book of Humorous Quotations.* New York, Dodd Mead, 1969:329.
17. Shiffman SM: The tobacco withdrawal syndrome, in Krasnegor NA (ed): *Cigarette Smoking as a Dependence Process* (NIDA Research Monograph 23). US Department of Health, Education, and Welfare, 1979.
18. Heimstra NW: The effects of smoking on mood change, in Dunn WL (ed): *Smoking Behavior: Motives and Incentives.* Washington, DC, Winston and Sons, 1973:197-207.
19. Perlick D: *The Withdrawal Syndrome: Nicotine Addiction and the Effects of Stopping Smoking in Heavy and Light Smokers* (thesis). Columbia University, New York, 1977.
20. Schachter S: Nicotine regulation in heavy and light smokers. *J Exp Psychol (Gen)* 1977;106:5-12.
21. Schwartz JL, Dubitzky M: Changes in anxiety, mood, and self-esteem resulting from an attempt to stop smoking. *Am J Psychiatry* 1968;124:138-142.
22. Kleinman KM, Vaugn RL, Christ TS: Effects of cigarette smoking and smoking deprivation on paired-associate learning of high and low meaningful nonsense syllables. *Psychol Rep* 1973;32:963-966.
23. Carney RM, Goldberg AP: Weight gain after cessation of cigarette smoking. *N Engl J Med* 1984;310:614-616.

24. Grunberg NE: The effects of nicotine and cigarette smoking on food consumption and taste preferences. *Addict Behav* 1982;7:317-331.
25. Soldatos CR, Kales JD, Scharf MB, Bixler EO, Kales A: Cigarette smoking associated with sleep difficulty. *Science* 1980;207:551-553.
26. Wack JT, Rodin J: Smoking and its effects on body weight and the systems of caloric regulation. *Am J Clin Nutr* 1982;35:366-380.
27. Glauser SC, Glauser EM, Reidenberg MM, Rusy BF, Tallarida RJ: Metabolic changes associated with the cessation of cigarette smoking. *Arch Environ Health* 1970;20:377-381.
28. Murphee HB, Schultz RE: Abstinence effects in smokers. *Fed Proc* 1968;27:220.
29. Ulett JA, Itil TM: Quantitative electroencephalogram in smoking and smoking deprivation. *Science* 1969;164:969-970.
30. Schachter S: Recidivism and self-cure of smoking and obesity. *Am Psychol* 1982;37:436-444.
31. Marlatt GA, Parks, GA: Self-management of addictive behaviors, in Karoly P, Kanfer FH (eds): *Self-Management and Behavior Change*. New York, Pergamon, 1982:443-488.
32. Meichenbaum D, Cameron R: Stress inoculation training, in Meichenbaum D, Jaremko ME (eds): *Stress Reduction and Prevention*. New York, Plenum, 1982:115-154.
33. Pechacek TF, Danaher BG: How and why people quit smoking: A cognitive-behavioral analysis, in Kendall PC, Hollon SD (eds): *Cognitive-Behavioral Interventions*. New York, Academic, 1979:389-422.
34. Shiffman S: Relapse following smoking cessation: A situational analysis. *J Consult Clin Psychol* 1982;50:71-86.
35. Mermelstein R, Lichtenstein E, McIntyre K: Partner support and relapse in smoking-cessation programs. *J Consult Clin Psychol* 1983;51:465-466.
36. Warrenburg S, Pagano RR, Woods M, Hlastala M: A comparison of somatic relaxation and EEG activity in classical progressive relaxation and transcendental meditation. *J Behav Med* 1980;3:73-93.
37. Roskies E: Stress management for Type A individuals, in Meichenbaum D, Jaremko ME (eds): *Stress Reduction and Prevention*. New York, Plenum, 1982:261-288.
38. Benson H: *The Relaxation Response*. New York, William Morrow, 1975.

39. Davis M, Eshelman ER, McKay M: *The Relaxation and Stress Reduction Workbook.* California, New Harbinger Publications, 1980.
40. McKay M, Davis M, Fanning P: *Thoughts and Feelings: The Art of Cognitive Stress Intervention.* California, New Harbinger Publications, 1981.
41. Little CC: Why do people think that quitting smoking affects their appetite or their weight? *Apothecary* 1964; Aug N-55.
42. Grunberg NE: Obesity: Etiology, hazards and treatment, in Gatchel RJ, Baum A, Singer JE (eds): *Handbook of Psychology and Health, Vol 1: Clinical Psychology and Behavioral Medicine: Overlapping Disciplines.* Hillsdale, NJ, Lawrence Erlbaum, 1982:103-119.
43. Powers PS: *Obesity, the Regulation of Weight.* Baltimore, Williams and Wilkins, 1980.
44. Stuart RB, Mitchell C, Jensen JA: Therapeutic options in the management of obesity, in Prokop CK, Bradley LA (eds): *Medical Psychology: Contributions to Behavioral Medicine.* New York, Academic, 1981:321-353.
45. Grunberg NE, Bowen DJ: Effects of nicotine on physical activity and body weight. Presented at the annual meeting of the American Psychological Association, Los Angeles, August 1983.
46. Grunberg NE, Bowen DJ, Morse DE: Effects of nicotine on body weight and food consumption in rats. *Psychopharmacology* 1984;83:93-98.
47. Grunberg NE, Morse DE: Cigarette smoking and food consumption in the United States. *J Appl Soc Psychol* 1984;14:310-317.

4

The Psychologic Effects of Exercise*

Donald Goff and Joel E. Dimsdale

INTRODUCTION

This chapter will discuss the evidence connecting exercise, primarily running, with psychologic well-being. This area of interest is not new; many cultural movements have embraced the ideal of physical and emotional perfection. During the 1850s, for example, Oliver Wendell Holmes, one of the leaders of the Muscular Christianity movement, advocated vigorous exercise as a means of developing emotional and moral health.[1]

In the past decade there has been a resurgence of enthusiasm for physical fitness and long-distance running. Record numbers of previously sedentary people now participate in vigorous physical fitness programs. The proliferation of books and magazines on running and the public fascination with marathon running illustrate this cultural trend. Recent studies polling large numbers of running enthusiasts show a fervently held conviction that running improves many aspects of psychologic function, especially mood, energy, and stress management.[2] Some studies also indicate that runners feel significant distress

---

*This work was supported by a Clinician Scientist Award from the American Heart Association with funds contributed by the Massachusetts heart affiliate and by grant HL31574 from the National Heart, Lung, and Blood Institute. Also, the authors are grateful to Drs. M. L. Sachs and J. H. Greist for advice on this chapter.

when forced to discontinue their running.[3] Similar beliefs are shared by a large part of the medical community; in one poll, 98% of physicians believed that running markedly improves psychologic as well as physical health.[4]

The subject of exercise and mental health is currently receiving growing attention from the mental health community, although much of the literature has not appeared in medical or psychiatric journals. A recent bibliography compiled by Sachs and Buffone listed over 1,000 references pertaining to the psychology of running and other forms of exercise.[5] Running has been offered as a therapy for a variety of psychiatric disorders, including depression,[6,7] anxiety states,[8] and phobias.[9-11] This new form of treatment, referred to by some as "jogotherapy,"[12] is being promoted by an international association of running therapists.

Although professionals and nonprofessionals believe that exercise makes people "feel better," few controlled studies have been performed to support the claims of those who prescribe it as a psychologic therapy. The issues are complex, since people exercise for many reasons and presumably experience diverse benefits. Some exercise for solitude, some out of gregariousness, some out of anger or anxiety, and some for a sense of mastery or control. Those who continue in the activity presumably experience a reinforcing psychologic effect that may be difficult to measure.

When psychologic benefits can be measured, they cannot be attributed solely to the exercise alone, since other factors are involved. One such factor is the expectation that exercise will yield psychologic benefits. This expectation is often imparted by zealous fitness instructors whose evangelical style "converts" the sedentary person into an exercise enthusiast. As Morgan pointed out in the case of runners, often many aspects of lifestyle change in conjunction with a regular running routine. Sorting out which psychologic effects are specific to the physical exertion, independent of other social, psychologic, or characterologic factors, is no small task.

ACUTE EXERCISE AND ANXIETY

Most of the attention on exercise and mental health has been directed towards the benefits of sustained physical conditioning. The immediate effects of a single period of exertion on anxiety and mood have been less well established,[12] although most runners report a vague sense of well-being after exercising. This post-exercise phenomenon is of practical importance, since the immediate reinforcement for running can enhance compliance with running programs.[13]

A number of studies have shown that brief vigorous exercise leads to a significant reduction in the frequency of self-reported anxiety and to changes in physiologic correlates of anxiety. De Vries used resting muscle electromyographic (EMG) activity as an indicator of stress.[14] After 15 minutes of vigorous exercise, a 58% reduction in resting action potential was demonstrated in a group of 29 college students. De Vries later compared exercise with meprobamate administration and concluded that exercise had the greater relaxant effect upon musculature.[15]

The degree of physical exertion appears to play a role in exercise-mediated stress reduction. Low-level exercise has only minimal beneficial effects on anxiety reduction.[16,17] More strenuous exercise is necessary for acute anxiety-diminishing effects. McPherson and colleagues[18] suggest that the level of fitness also contributes to the reduction of stress. In their study, regular exercisers, when compared with beginning exercisers, reported a significantly greater reduction of anxiety following a single period of exercise. This difference disappeared 20 weeks into the study, at which time the fitness level of the beginning exercisers had caught up with that of regular exercisers. These findings tend to corroborate the experience of many runners who report that the more vigorous the run, the greater the sense of well-being, and maintain that running when the participant is "out of shape" is much less rewarding than it is when the person is "in shape."

A recent study by Bahrke and Morgan[19] challenges the notion that the anxiety-reducing effect is directly attributable to acute exercise. Seventy-five regular exercisers were randomly assigned to a session of vigorous exercise, meditation, or 20 minutes of quiet rest with a copy of *Reader's Digest*. A similar and significant reduction in anxiety was found in each of the three groups. Whether this finding reflects the lack of specificity of the running effect or the insensitivity of anxiety scales remains to be determined. In a related study, Sime[17] evaluated the effects of exercise, meditation, and a placebo tranquilizer pill upon a number of psychologic measures of anxiety. Acute exercise was found to be superior to meditation and placebo for decreasing pulse rate and electrodermal response, but it was no better than the other two conditions in lowering resting blood pressure and EMG activity (frontalis muscle).

THE PSYCHOLOGIC EFFECTS OF SUSTAINED EXERCISE PROGRAMS

A large number of studies have attempted to evaluate the effects of sustained physical conditioning on mood and personality. Many of these studies have simply measured aspects of mood and personality in runners and nonexercisers or participants in other sports. Runners have generally been found to be less depressed, less tense, and more self-confident than nonrunners.[20,21] The obvious objection to these studies is that exercise may not contribute to these differences in personality characteristics, but rather these personality characteristics may attract a person to running and possibly help sustain the interest; prospective studies have largely supported this objection. In a series of controlled studies, the effects of training programs on personality measures have been relatively small, with the exception of improvement in self-concept (variables such as body image and physical ability).[22-28] It should be noted, however, that Cattell's 16-Factor Personality Questionnaire has been the instrument used in most studies. This scale measures qualities such as intelligence and temperament, which are personality characteristics considered less likely to change in reaction to events or interventions.[29]

Recently, investigators have looked at different aspects of personality in relation to exercise. Using the Jenkins Activity Survey (JAS) as a measure of Type A personality, Blumenthal and colleagues[30] demonstrated that Type A individuals could significantly reduce their JAS score after a 10-week exercise program. Lobitz and co-workers[31] further examined this effect by assigning subjects to a 7-week program of anxiety management training, physical exercise, or no treatment. They found that JAS Type A scores were reduced by exercise for all subjects, whereas anxiety management training did not significantly reduce JAS scores.[31,32] The reason for the beneficial effect of exercise on Type A traits has not been clarified, though it has been suggested that Type A is a pattern of coping with uncontrollable stress, and thus, Type A people may derive particular benefit from the sense of mastery and control afforded by the completion of an exercise program.[33] This area of research remains preliminary, but is of interest in light of the studies examining the relationship of Type A traits to cardiovascular disease.[34,35]

Although fitness programs do not appear to affect most aspects of personality, they do bring about an improvement in mood.[36-39] Most of the literature on this subject is composed of poorly controlled studies comparing populations biased because of self-selection. For instance, enrollees in fitness classes, who expect physical and emotional benefit, are frequently compared with nonexercisers. A few of the better controlled studies will be described below, since the findings may shed some light on who benefits from exercise and why.

Greist and co-workers[40] performed one of the first controlled trials of running therapy by randomly assigning 28 patients with minor depression to programs of exercise, time-limited psychotherapy, or time-unlimited psychotherapy. At the end of 12 weeks, the improvement in depression of the running group was roughly equal to that of the time-limited psychotherapy group and superior to that of the time-unlimited psychotherapy group. Statistical analysis was not done because of the small sample size. A subsequent attempt by the same researchers to repeat the study with a larger patient population assigned to group running, group psychotherapy, or meditation was unsuccessful owing to a staggering dropout rate. Of the first 30 subjects, 75% of runners, 50% of meditators, and 40% of group therapy participants terminated before completing the program.[41] When Greist and associates returned to the study design using an individual running therapist, the 75% dropout rate recorded for the running group was reduced to 20%. These results are of particular interest because they demonstrate the difficulty of assigning such treatments to depressed patients and emphasize the significance of the individual contact with the therapist in running therapy. Compliance is much better with an enthusiastic individual instructor than with an instructor in a group setting. For many participants, the psychologic benefits may result as much from the relationship with an individual running companion as from the activity of running.

Folkins[42] evaluated the effects of physical conditioning on 40 policemen and firemen selected on the basis of elevated coronary risk factors. Subjects were assigned by matched pairing to either an exercise group or a control group. After 12 weeks of exercise (three sessions per week), the exercise group showed significant improvement in all levels of cardiovascular fitness, decreases in measures of anxiety ($P < .01$), and decreases in depression scores ($P < .05$). These results are more impressive than those of many other controlled studies, probably because of the high rate of compliance with exercise. This study was also one of the few in which control subjects agreed to refrain from exercise, thus highlighting the difference between groups.

A second study by Folkins, although less well controlled, is of interest in that it addresses the question of who benefits most from conditioning.[43] The authors compared 84 college students who had enrolled in a 12-week course of jogging, archery, or golf. Although the men and women in the jogging class improved their fitness, only the women joggers showed significant improvement in levels of anxiety, depression, and self-confidence. Further analysis revealed that prior to beginning the program, the female joggers were significantly less fit than the men, and more anxious, depressed, and less confident than the men or women in the other sports groups. This study demonstrates a potential flaw of studies that do not use random assignment - subjects who choose to enroll in running programs may be quite different from controls. In fact, some studies suggest a higher frequency of affective disorders in runners, particularly in women.[44] The study also suggests a tendency for the least fit and the most anxious or depressed to reap the greatest benefit from conditioning programs *if* they comply with the exercise program.

PSYCHOLOGIC EFFECTS OF CARDIAC REHABILITATION

Some of the most extensive work on exercise and psychologic health comes from studies of rehabilitation programs for patients suffering a myocardial infarction (MI). This event threatens one's self-concept of being strong, successful, and invulnerable; as a result, depression and anxiety are common complications.[45,46] For this reason, investigators in cardiac rehabilitation settings have paid particular attention to controlling for factors nonspecific to running, since post-MI patients are more apt to benefit from any activity that lessens their sense of physical and social impairment.

The significance of depression after MI is highlighted by a study reported by Kavanaugh and colleagues.[47] Forty-four subjects with scores of depression greater than 70 (assessed by the Minnesota Multiphasic Personality Inventory) were selected from a group of 100 patients post-MI. The subjects were then enrolled in a program of exercise three times per week and were evaluated after 4 years. Collectively, the subjects had a significant decrease in depression scores ($P < .001$), yet 50% of the subjects continued to have a depression score greater than two standard deviations above the normal. Improvement in depression score did not correlate with improved cardiovascular fitness but was strongly correlated with compliance; only those subjects who attended a minimum of 60% of exercise sessions reported a reduction in depression score. In addition to demonstrating the severity and chronicity of depressed mood after infarction, this study also raises the question of how compliance is associated with the antidepressant effect of exercise. The correlation between compliance and antidepressant effect can be viewed either as evidence that most subjects improve if they stick with the exercise program or as evidence that many subjects remain depressed despite exercising and hence become noncompliant with a treatment that is perceived as unhelpful.

An earlier study by McPherson and associates[18] helps sort out some nonspecific effects of exercise programs in cardiac rehabilitation. Men with MI and healthy controls were assigned by matched pairing either to a twice-weekly program of graduated exercise or to a control group that met once weekly for recreational swimming. Before the program was begun, personality tests were administered and revealed the cardiac patients to be more tense, aloof, and aggressive than the healthy subjects. At the end of 24 weeks, the post-infarction patients showed significant improvement in mood, anxiety, and sense of well-being; those who exercised were most improved on a majority of scales. In contrast, the control group of non-cardiac subjects did not show benefits from the exercise program. The dramatic increase in sense of well-being achieved by the cardiac exercisers is impressive, but of equal interest is the significant improvement that the recreational swimmers enjoyed without achieving significant improvement in physical fitness. The nonspecific effects of mobilizing post-infarction patients who are apprehensive about physical activity and engaging them in a social activity appear to be a powerful factor in the success of cardiac rehabilitation, independent of physical fitness.

An important contribution to the field was provided in Stern and Cleary's psychologic evaluation of participants in the National Exercise and Heart Disease Project.[48,49] In this study, 784 post-MI men were assigned either to an exercise program or to a control group. Prior to random assignment, all subjects participated in a 6-week, low-level exercise program designed to weed out those who were noncompliant. Fifteen percent of the subjects dropped out during this interval; dropouts tended to be of lower socioeconomic level, had fewer previous MIs, and were significantly longer post-infarction than nondropouts. Dropouts also reported higher anxiety, depression, and stress, and were rated by spouses as having more psychopathology. For subjects who completed the initial 6-week program, significant improvements in depression, vocational activity, and sexual function were recorded.

In phase 2 of the study, the subjects were assigned to exercise or control groups. The exercise group was urged to attend three 45-minute sessions per week of activity designed to allow them to achieve 70% to 80% of their age-predicted maximum heart rate. During the first 2 months, 90% of exercisers attended at least 90% of the sessions; however, by month 18, only 48% of subjects were attending >50% of the sessions. Interestingly, and perhaps disastrously for the research comparison, by month 18, 30% of control subjects reported exercising independently on a regular basis. With few exceptions, a battery of psychologic measures failed to show any difference between exercisers and controls in mood, anxiety, adjustment, and locus of control at any point during the 2-year follow-up.

Like the findings of McPherson and associates,[18] these results show the significant benefits produced by low-level, short-term exercise programs for post-MI patients. The failure to document any further psychologic benefits from a 2-year program is intriguing and amenable to many possible explanations. First, compliance is a factor; it is very difficult to maintain an adequate difference in activity levels between controls and experimental subjects over a period of years. Second, detecting an improvement in psychologic measures may become increasingly difficult after the most depressed and anxious subjects have dropped out. Stern and Cleary raise a final point in noting that some subjects complained of feeling "washed out" after exercise sessions and reported a worsening of their psychologic state as a result of the exercise program. This negative response to vigorous exercise in some subjects might be masking the cumulative benefit experienced by the majority of participants.

CONCLUSION

Clearly, many people experience improved mood and self-esteem associated with exercise; however, we are probably not all "born to jog." The potential psychologic gain from exercise and the likelihood of sustaining the activity may both be largely determined by an individual's physical and characterologic make-up.

For many people, especially cardiac patients, long-term vigorous exercise programs do not add significant advantage over low-level, short-term activities such as recreational swimming. Similarly, the relaxant effect of single exercise sessions can be equaled by meditation or by rest.

Greater physical fitness does enhance the positive reinforcement gained from individual exercise sessions, but also predisposes the subject to withdrawal distress when regular exercise is interrupted. On the other hand, poorly conditioned subjects show the greatest psychologic improvements in sustained conditioning programs.

The effects of intensive running programs are less clear, since few studies have randomly assigned subjects to such training. Because long-distance runners and their sedentary counterparts differ significantly on many psychologic variables, uncontrolled studies comparing the two groups are not helpful.

As the study by Stern and Cleary illustrates, over an extended period of time, control and experimental groups begin to resemble each other in their exercise levels, thus decreasing the difference between the groups. When studies report large dropout rates with the remaining subjects showing greater psychologic gain, the tendency is to attribute the gain to the level of participation (the "dose" of exercise). However, an alternate explanation is that those who drop out do so because they were not benefiting from the exercise.

A small number of studies have begun to address the psychologic effects of exercise in scientific fashion. Additional studies are needed that would use random assignment to documented exercise and control programs. We do not yet understand the determinants of who benefits from exercise or how to maximize the positive effects. As evidence accumulates supporting the connection between exercise and psychologic functioning, more attention will have to be focused on methods of improving compliance. Meanwhile, physical exercise should be encouraged for its associated benefits of enhanced sense of personal achievement and social participation.

REFERENCES

1. Lucas JA, Smith RA: *Saga of American Sport.* Philadelphia, Lea and Febiger, 1978.
2. Harris MB: Runners' perceptions of the benefits of running. *Percept Mot Skills* 1981;52:153-154.
3. Baekeland F: Exercise deprivation: Sleep and psychological reactions. *Arch Gen Psychiatry* 1970;22:365-369.
4. Byrd OE: The relief of tension by exercise: A survey of medical viewpoints and practices. *J Sch Health* 1963;33:238-239.
5. Sachs ML, Buffone GW: *Bibliography: Psychological Considerations in Exercise, Including Exercise as Psychotherapy, Exercise Dependence (Exercise Addiction) and the Psychology of Running.* (Unpublished).
6. Blue FR: Aerobic running as a treatment for moderate depression (abstract). *Percept Mot Skills* 1979;48:228.
7. Brown RS, Ramirez DE, Taub JM: The prescription of exercise for depression. *Physician and Sportsmedicine* 1978;6:34-45.
8. Driscoll R: Anxiety reduction using physical exertion and positive images. *Psychol Record* 1976;26:87-94.
9. Muller B, Armstrong HE: A further note on the "running treatment" for anxiety. *Psychotherapy: Theory, Research, Practice* 1975;12:385-387.
10. Orwin A: The running treatment: A preliminary communication of a new use for an old therapy (physical activity) in the agoraphobic syndrome. *Br J Psychiatry* 1973;122:175-179.
11. Orwin A: Treatment of a situational phobia-A case for running. *Br J Psychiatry* 1974;125:95-98.
12. Harper FD: *Jogotherapy: Jogging as a therapeutic strategy.* Alexandria, VA, Douglas Publishers, 1979.

13. Sachs ML: Compliance and addiction to exercise, in Cantu RC (ed): *The Exercising Adult*. Lexington, MA, The Collamore Press, 1982:19-27.
14. de Vries HA: Immediate and long-term effects of exercise upon resting muscle action potential level. *J Sports Med Phys Fitness* 1968;8:1-11.
15. de Vries HA, Adams GM: Electromyographic comparison of single dose of exercise and meprobamate as to effects on muscular relaxation. *Am J Phys Med* 1972;51: 130-141.
16. Morgan WP, Roberts JA, Feinerman AD: Psychologic effect of acute physical activity. *Arch Phys Med Rehabil* 1971;52:422-425.
17. Sime WE: A comparison of exercise and meditation in reducing physiological response to stress (abstract). *Med Sci Sports Exerc* 1977;9:55.
18. McPherson BD, Paivio A, Yuhasz MS, Rechnitzer PA, Pickard H, Lefcoe N: Psychological effects of an exercise program for post infarct and normal adult men. *J Sports Med Phys Fitness* 1965;8:95-102.
19. Bahrke MS, Morgan WP: Anxiety reduction following exercise and meditation. *Cognitive Therapy and Research* 1978;2:323-334.
20. Morgan WP, Pollock ML: Psychologic characterization of the elite distance runner. *Ann NY Acad Sci* 1977;301:382-402.
21. Gondola JC, Tuckman BW: Psychological mood state in "average" marathon runners. *Percept Mot Skills* 1982; 55:1295-1300.
22. Buccola VA, Stone WJ: Effects of jogging and cycling programs on physiological and personality variables in aged men. *Research Quarterly* 1975;46:134-139.
23. Collingswood TR: The effects of physical training upon behavior and self attitudes. *J Clin Psychol* 1972; 28:583-585.
24. Folkins CH, Sime WE: Physical fitness training and mental health. *Am Psychol* 1981;36:373-389.
25. Gary V, Guthrie D: The effect of jogging on physical fitness and self concept in hospitalized alcoholics. *Quarterly Journal of Studies on Alcohol* 1972;33:1073-1078.
26. Layman EM: Psychological effects of physical activity, in Wilmore JH (ed): *Exercise and Sports Sciences Reviews*. New York, Academic Press, 1974:33-70.
27. Hilyer J, Mitchell W: Effect of systematic physical fitness training combined with counseling on the self con-

cept of college students. *J Counselling Psychol* 1979; 26:427-436.
28. McGowan RW, Jarman BO, Pederson DM: Effects of a competitive endurance training program on self-concept and peer approval. *J Psychol* 1974;86:57-60.
29. Cattell RB, Eber HW, Tatsuoka MM: *Handbook for the Sixteen Personality Factor Questionnaire in Clinical, Educational, Industrial and Research Psychology.* Champaign, IL, Institute for Personality and Ability Testing, 1970.
30. Blumenthal JA, Williams RS, Williams RB, Wallace AG: Effects of exercise on the type A (coronary prone) behavior pattern. *Psychosom Med* 1980;42:289-296.
31. Lobitz CW, Brammell HL, Stoll S, Niccoli A: Physical exercise and anxiety management training for cardiac stress management in a nonpatient population. *J Cardiac Rehabil* 1983;3:683-688.
32. Blumenthal JA, Williams RS, Williams AG: Psychological changes accompanying physical exercise: A controlled study (abstract). *Psychosom Med* 1981;13:74.
33. Glass DC: Stress, behavior patterns and coronary disease. *Am Sci* 1977;65:177-187.
34. Jenkins CD, Rosenman RH, Zyzanski SJ: Prediction of clinical coronary heart disease by a test for the coronary-prone behavior pattern. *N Engl J Med* 1974;290:1271-1275.
35. Rosenman RH, Brand RJ, Jenkins CD, Friedman M, Strauss R, Wurm M: Coronary heart disease in the Western Collaborative Group study: Final follow-up experience of 8 1/2 years. *JAMA* 1975;233:872-877.
36. Folkins CH, Amsterdam EA: Control and modification of stress emotions through chronic exercise, in Amsterdam EA, Wilmore JH, Demaria AN (eds): *Exercise and Cardiovascular Health and Disease.* New York, Yorke Medical Books 1977:280-294.
37. Kowal DM, Patton JF, Vogel JA: Psychological states and aerobic fitness of male and female recruits before and after basic training. *Aviat Space Environ Med* 1978; 49:603-606.
38. Carter R: Exercise and happiness. *J Sports Med Phys Fitness* 1977;17:307-313.
39. Snyder EE, Spreitzer EA: Involvement in sports and psychological well-being. *International Journal of Sports Psychology* 1974; 5:28-39.
40. Greist JH, Klein MH, Eischens RR, Faris JT, Gurman AS, Morgan W: Running as treatment for depression. *Compr Psychiatry* 1979;20:41-54.

41. Greist JH, Eischens RR, Klein MH, Linn D: Addendum to "running through your mind," in Sacks MH, Sachs ML (eds): *Psychology of Running*. Champaign, IL, Human Kinetics Publishers, 1981:27-31.
42. Folkins CH: Effects of physical training on mood. *J Clin Psychol* 1976;32:385-388.
43. Folkins CH, Lynch S, Gradner MM: Psychological fitness as a function of physical fitness. *Arch Phys Med Rehabil* 1972;53:503-508.
44. Colt EWD, Dunner DL, Hall K, Fieve RR: A high prevalence of affective disorders in runners, in Sacks MH, Sachs ML (eds): *Psychology of Running*. Champaign, IL, Human Kinetics Publishers, 1981.
45. Hellerstein HK, Ford AB: Rehabilitation of the cardiac patient. *JAMA* 1957;164:225-231.
46. Wishnie HA, Hackett TP, Cassem NH: Psychological hazards of convalescence following myocardial infarction. *JAMA* 1971;215:1292-1296.
47. Kavanaugh T, Shephard RJ, Tuck JAA, Qureshi S: Depression following myocardial infarction: The effect of distance running. *Ann NY Acad Sci* 1977;301:1029-1038.
48. Stern MJ, Cleary P: National exercise and heart disease project. Psychosocial changes observed during a low-level exercise program. *Arch Intern Med* 1981;141:1463-1467.
49. Stern MJ, Cleary P: National exercise and heart disease project. Long-term psychosocial outcome. *Arch Intern Med* 1982;142:1093-1097.

5

Psychiatric Management of the Hospitalized Cardiac Patient*

George E. Tesar and Thomas P. Hackett

INTRODUCTION

The psychologic response of patients to cardiac illness has stimulated interest and research among physicians, psychologists, nurses, and social workers for the last three decades. This is due in part to the unique qualities of cardiac patients and their experience. The typical patient is a man who is a provider at the helm of his career and family; he has often been active and in relatively good health prior to the unexpected manifestation of disease. Cardiac illness or the surgical treatment of it, therefore, may thrust the person suddenly and dramatically into an unfamiliar realm of disability and life-threatening symptoms. Compounding the stress of the illness itself is an increasing number of diagnostic tests and therapeutic interventions to which patients are subjected, such as cardiac catheterization, angioplasty, and electrophysiologic studies.

It is only natural, then, to wonder how the patient copes with the emotional ordeal of acute cardiac illness. In fact, over time, most patients do quite well, as demonstrated by studies of post-surgical[1] and post-myocardial infarction (MI)[2] patients. During the acute phase of illness, the majority of patients adapt well to the illness and its treatment.[3-5] Nevertheless, most suffer psychiatric

---

*The authors wish to thank Ned H. Cassem, MD, for his helpful comments and assistance in preparation of this chapter.

sequelae that necessitate additional specific treatment.[6] The purpose of this chapter is to outline these problems and to discuss their evaluation and management.

CORONARY CARE UNIT

Patients admitted to a coronary care unit (CCU) have a predictable sequence of emotional reactions, including anxiety, denial, despondency, and manifestation of chronic personality traits.[6] These reactions are expected responses to stressful circumstances and generally do not require the intervention of a specialist. However, if a patient's reactions do not receive sufficient attention, or if they exceed the management capabilities of the primary care physician, then referral to a specialist will be necessary.[6]

ANXIETY

Most cardiac patients will be admitted to the CCU via the hospital's emergency room, and in large tertiary-care hospitals, many visit the cardiac catheterization laboratory for study just prior to arrival in the CCU. Emotionally aroused by these events, patients are then introduced to a new environment outfitted with unfamiliar monitoring and therapeutic equipment, including a cardiac monitor, intravenous bottles and lines, oxygen administration equipment, and in extreme cases a mechanical ventilator, an intra-aortic balloon pump, or both. Anxiety may be further stimulated by pain, discomfort, the ever-present threat of death, or even identification with a significant other whose cause of death was MI. Experiencing cardiac arrest might be expected to further increase anxiety and general psychiatric morbidity, but this has not been found to be the case.[5]

Treatment. Familiarizing the patient with the CCU - its machinery, protocol, and restrictions - is a vital first step in allaying anxiety, but one must also take pains to insure that the information delivered is being received and processed. Out of bewilderment, anxiety, and possibly confusion, new patients are often minimally attentive; consequently, orienting information may have to be repeated more than once.

Human contact,[7] appropriate reassurance, instruction, clarification, and opportunity for ventilation are vital instruments that can reduce a patient's anxiety.[8] Often patients are not immediately receptive to caring and empathic efforts. Some require encouragement to open up, and some will simply fail to ask about areas of concern to them; questions about death, prognosis, and discomfort can be anticipated and raised by physicians for such patients.[9]

Pharmacologic treatment of anxiety should be instituted in all patients, particularly in those who manifest heightened autonomic responses to stressful stimuli (alarm bells, physicians on rounds, etc.).[8] Diazepam 5-10 mg orally q8h is still the most effective tranquilizing agent, primarily because of its potency and duration of action; it should be ordered on a regular basis, not prn, since not all patients who need medication request it.[8] Morphine sulfate, effective in the management of infarction pain, also has a concomitant anxiolytic effect.[8] If hepatic metabolism is impaired by age, congestion, or primary hepatic insufficiency, suitable alternative oral agents are lorazepam 1-2 mg q8H or oxazepam 15-30 mg q4h, both of which are excreted exclusively by the kidneys.

If anxiety persists or cannot be allayed, consultation will be necessary. Anger, fear of sedation, insufficient pharmacologic treatment, and psychotic denial are factors that may render first-line management efforts ineffective.[6] Use of an antipsychotic agent may be necessary in cases of intense anxiety not controlled by mild tranquilizers.

DENIAL

Denial is defined as "the conscious or unconscious repudiation of all or a portion of the total available meaning of an illness in order to allay anxiety and to minimize emotional stress."[10] This defense mechanism is believed to play a role in keeping the MI patient's affective responses in check.[10] Patients who use denial in this way cope by denying or minimizing their fear. This must be distinguished from an alternative use of denial in which the reality and gravity of illness are rejected. Confusion of these two uses of denial leads to misunderstanding of the concept as it relates to cardiac illness.

Denial of illness is maladaptive and a precursor to noncompliance. It is also an ineffective means of coping with anxiety, for the anxiety is inevitably rechanneled and expressed as anger or depression. The patient who uses denial adaptively will accept the fact and implications of his or her illness, but deny fear of its consequences - "When my time comes, I'll be ready." Of course, such a remark may be used to mask underlying anxiety, but such efforts will usually be betrayed by objective signs of discomfort: palmar sweating, rigid/fixed countenance, and so on.[10]

Treatment. Those who deny the fact as well as the impact of their illness create potential management problems. A concerted effort must be made to elicit the patient's cooperation. Repeated efforts to convince him or her of the facts are generally unproductive, if not inflammatory. If this approach fails, extra sedative oral medication or a neuroleptic, such as thiothixene or haloperidol 5 mg bid, may be necessary to alleviate the anxiety that stimulates maladaptive denial.

DEPRESSION

As anxiety and denial diminish, the patient begins to assimilate the events of the preceding days. Many will respond to the realization of their newly acquired infirmity and disability with sadness and a sense of loss, the significance of which varies from individual to individual. It can be said that the typical patient suffers an "infarction of the ego" as well as the myocardium.[6] The sudden loss of power and potential stands in marked contrast to the prowess and productivity experienced by many patients prior to their MI. The experience of loss is exacerbated by pre-existing depression, other life stresses, and by myths about the implications of an MI.[6]

Treatment. Generally, the depression experienced by CCU patients is transient, responds to brief supportive psychotherapy, and does not require treatment with antidepressant medication.[6] Ventilation and discussion are useful in relieving the despondency and sense of helplessness that may be experienced. Misconceptions should be dispelled; the patient should be informed that weakness can be expected both now and to a lesser extent in the future, during recuperation.[6] The patient should also be given the opportunity to discuss financial and domestic problems, which are often high in the hierarchy of patient concerns.[9]

PERSONALITY AND BEHAVIORAL DISTURBANCES

Under stress, susceptible individuals may regress to more primitive methods of coping. Psychotic denial, passive-aggressive acting-out, sexual provocativeness, and outright refusal to comply with treatment are defense mechanisms commonly observed.[8] Patients with pre-existing personality disorders (narcissistic and borderline) are most likely to create disturbances;[11] however, male patients with adequate premorbid personalities who have sustained a significant ego infarction (i.e., they feel "less than a man"[6]) may attempt to reinforce their masculinity by behaving in a provocative and sexually aggressive fashion. Similarly, the injury to self-esteem may provoke anger, resulting in noncompliance or withdrawal.

In addition, individuals with Type A personality characteristics (see Chapter 7) may cause disturbance with their impatience, need for control, and intolerance of limitations. However, the response of Type A individuals to the CCU has not been widely investigated.[12] One study[13] suggests that these individuals may actually adapt quite well through their employment of denial and a positive attitude.

Treatment. Supportive psychotherapy can be helpful, but unless it is used with discretion, it will be ineffective and may aggravate these problems. If acting-out occurs in response to feeling isolated and misunderstood, then establishment of empathic contact is important. Requesting the patient's cooperation can also be helpful. Some patients may not agree with the treatment prescribed, but nevertheless may comply if it is made clear to them that their cooperation will improve the care they receive.[11]

If other techniques fail, the problem patient must be confronted and strict limits enforced.[8] Confrontation is an invaluable method, but must be used without anger. Though patients may not be aware of their behavior or its impact, once the behavior is acknowledged, it can be observed and altered.

The patient who threatens to sign out against medical advice is an irksome but uncommon problem. Baile and co-workers[14] identified only 2% who signed out during a 3-year period of observation. Such individuals were characterized by younger age, relatively less severe medical problems, histories of alcoholism, previous signouts against medical advice, and personality disturbances. Intervention techniques include reassurance, clarification of misconceptions, and evaluation for and treatment of psychosis.[6,14]

DELIRIUM

Delirium has been reported to occur in 3% to 10% of patients in the CCU.[5,12] Any one of a number of factors peculiar to the CCU may precipitate a delirium, and delirium is often of multifactorial etiology, which accounts for its variable presentation. Characteristically, confusion and paranoia are manifested by behavioral reactions ranging from restlessness and irritability to hostility, belligerence, and combativeness that may be dangerous to both staff and patient. Some disorientation is usually present, but the degree and duration may vary over 24 hours. Visual hallucinations suggest a toxic or metabolic etiology.

The determinants of delirium in the CCU include (a) environmental factors such as monotony, noise, and confinement; (b) metabolic disturbances; (c) drugs; (d) withdrawal states; (e) sleep deprivation; and (f) factors peculiar to the individual, such as age, level of anxiety, general state of health, pre-existing central nervous system dysfunction, and possibly maladaptive personality traits.[15] The etiologic significance of environmental factors has been emphasized,[15-17] but other patients exposed to the same environmental circumstances tolerate them well, which suggests that the simultaneous occurrence of other precipitants is necessary.[18]

Evaluation of the agitated/delirious patient should include consideration of the principles outlined in Table 1 (page 73).

Treatment. Treatment involves (a) correction of metabolic and systemic abnormalities, (b) elimination or alteration of medications producing toxicity, (c) treatment of withdrawal states, and (d) use of neuroleptic medication.[19] Maximization of the patient's physical comfort, attention to his or her emotional needs, and the physical presence of the nurse, physician, or family are important measures but not always practical, and are insufficient to control the increasing agitation of the confused and paranoid patient. In such cases, pharmacologic treatment and sometimes physical restraints are indicated for the safety and comfort of patient and staff.

TABLE 1: EVALUATION OF DELIRIUM IN THE INTENSIVE CARE UNIT

Etiologic and Predisposing Factors	Check
Previous delirium or psychosis	History
Cardiac arrest	History
Use of drugs, alcohol, and cigarettes	History
Respiratory disturbance	Arterial blood gas levels
Fluid and electrolyte imbalance	Osmolarity, serum electrolytes
Hemodynamic impairment	BP, cardiac index, carotid arteries, ECG
Hypoglycemia	Blood sugar levels
Thyroid dysfunction	Thyroid function tests
Fever/infection	Temperature, cultures
CNS dysfunction	History, LP, EEG, CT scan, VDRL
Anemia	CBC
Hepatic insufficiency	Liver function tests, serum ammonia
Renal insufficiency	BUN/creatinine levels
Withdrawal states (drugs, alcohol)	History
Toxins: cimetidine, digitalis, lidocaine	Visual hallucinations, slurred speech, toxic screen

BP = blood pressure; ECG = electrocardiogram; CNS - central nervous system; LP = lumbar puncture, EEG = electroencephalogram; CT = computed tomographic; VDRL - venereal disease reaction level; CBC = complete blood count; BUN = blood urea nitrogen.

Haloperidol is the medication of choice.[19,20] Starting doses of 2-10 mg have been advocated and in most instances will be sufficient to initiate control, but larger doses may be necessary to subdue certain patients.[20] We have cared for patients, most of them receiving intraaortic balloon counterpulsation, who have required large doses of intravenous haloperidol - as high as 300-400 mg during a 24-hour period - to control severe agitation (unpublished data). Maintenance dosage and interval of administration are determined by the degree of subsequent agitation. At present, intravenous administration of haloperidol can only be used as an "innovative" therapy; however, it is remarkably safe and effective, producing little if any akathisia or dystonia compared with oral or intramuscular administration.[20] When hypotension results, it is invariably related to the presence of other factors, such as decreased systemic vascular resistance and hypovolemia.

SLEEP-CYCLE DEFECTS

The sleep-wake cycle and its electroencephalographic (EEG) correlates are markedly impaired in post-MI patients.[6,21] Many patients will experience fragmented sleep at night and prolongation of daytime sleep. The sleep-EEG demonstrates absence of stages 3 and 4 sleep and marked reduction of rapid eye movement sleep. Practically speaking, this means that the patient never achieves a state of deep sleep. This has been thought to predispose to delirium[19] and is associated with a peak in episodes of nocturnal angina on nights 4 and 5 after MI,[6] although there is no association between ischemic episodes and sleep stages.[21] Normalization of the sleep pattern occurs approximately at day 9 after MI.[6]

Treatment. Some patients stay awake because of the fear that they will die during sleep. Anticipation of this concern and reassurance are often helpful.

Use of benzodiazepines for sedation is advised.[5,6,8,21] Several potent hypnotics with short half-lives are available to induce nocturnal sleep: oral lorazepam 2-4 mg, oral temazepam 15-30 mg, oral alprazolam 0.5-1.0 mg, and oral triazolam 0.25-0.5 mg. Oxazepam is relatively ineffective as a hypnotic for many patients.

FAMILIAL FACTORS

Families struggle with the same issues that afflict patients. From their vantage point as observers, family members may feel helpless to do anything constructive, or may overestimate the degree to which the patient is suffering.

Treatment. Families need to be talked with, oriented, reassured, and even confronted when their behaviors exceed appropriate limits. It is helpful to have regular meetings in which family members can ask questions and share concerns;[8] this may be done with individual or multiple families. It is often useful to designate one member as spokesman with large families. Occasionally, a family member will request medication for "nerves." The cause for concern should be identified and discussed, but requests for medication should be discouraged and, if necessary, referred elsewhere.

TRANSFER FROM THE CCU

This step is regarded by most patients as evidence of improvement and progress, and they are reassured by their graduation.[5] Some patients, though, experience the move as a loss of support, both mechanical and human. In these patients the transition may be associated with elevations of catecholamines and subsequent complications.[22] Patients requiring greater surveillance and attention are those who are single, those who have become particularly attached to the CCU and its staff, and those who have a history of intense or unmet dependency needs.

Treatment. Patients leaving the CCU should be prepared in advance for their transfer. Individuals susceptible to the effects of separation should be identified and extra attention paid to their preparation. If possible, one or more of the CCU staff should pay such patients a follow-up visit for the sake of continuity.[22]

CARDIAC SURGERY

Over the past 15 to 20 years, investigations of the psychologic impact of cardiac surgery have concentrated primarily on the etiology, prevention, recognition, and treatment of post-operative delirium. Long-term psychologic outcome after cardiac surgery is good,[1] indicating that the occurrence of post-operative delirium is a circumscribed problem without long-term consequences. It is, however, a common problem, occurring in one-sixth to one-third of patients,[15,17] and is taxing and painful for both health care professionals and patients.

Post-operative delirium is not fundamentally different from delirium occurring in any intensive care unit, except for the addition of determinants related to the cardiac surgery itself. The frequency of delirium after cardiac surgery varies according to the type of procedure performed. Most studies have examined the phenomenon following cardiotomy (open-heart surgery).[15] Here, the incidence has been reported to be anywhere from 22% to 57%,[15] whereas following coronary artery bypass graft surgery (CABGS), the incidence is 13% to 28%.[17,23] This contrasts with a 0.1% incidence of post-operative delirium in the general surgical population.[24] The incidence data for delirium after cardiac surgery are based on procedures performed before 1975. Therefore, with improved surgical techniques, and particularly with the replacement of the disk by the bubble oxygenator, the current incidence of delirium is probably even lower.

It is useful to divide etiologic factors into those occurring in the pre-operative phase, those occurring in the operative phase, and those occurring in the post-operative phase. Probably the most important pre-operative factors that cause delirium are severity of physical illness and presence of central nervous system disease.[15,25] Among the other predictors are the patient's flexibility and durability in dealing with stressful circumstances.[26] Though a uniform psychologic profile has not been associated with post-cardiotomy delirium,[15] some correlation has been reported in patients who manifest significant pre-operative anxiety, depression, and rejection of the planned procedure,[23] and the incidence appears to decrease in patients who demonstrate confidence and self-assurance.[17] Poor comprehension of the procedure, possibly due to denial, may also be a predictor of post-operative delirium.[23] Cardiac status,[25] including a history of MI,[17] has been associated with increased risk of both post-cardiotomy[15] and post-CABGS[17] delirium. Age and sex do not seem to have a consistent effect on outcome.[15]

Operative factors favoring onset of delirium following cardiotomy, though not necessarily following CABGS, include complexity of the surgical procedure, total anesthesia time, degree of hypothermia ($\leq 27°C$) and occurrence of intraoperative hypotension (systolic blood pressure <50-60 mm Hg).[15] Time on a heart-lung machine does not have any direct influence on outcome of either cardiotomy[15] or CABGS.[17]

Post-operative factors include features peculiar to the recovery room environment, for example, noise and monotony,[15,17,26] severity of recovery room illness,[17] and drugs administered, particularly those with anticholinergic properties.[27]

PREVENTION AND TREATMENT OF POST-OPERATIVE DELIRIUM

Though the effects of pre-operative intervention have not been proven successful, studies suggest that pre-operative teaching and preparation of the patient is valuable.[23] Pre-operative psychiatric interviews may also be helpful, but only if they are conducted on more than one occasion.[24] These studies[23,24] suggest that specific psychiatric attention should be paid to patients who have pre-operative anxiety or depression or who refuse surgery.

In the recovery room, it is important to consider all factors listed in Table 1 with a view to identifying and treating correctable abnormalities. The principles of treatment with neuroleptic agents are the same as discussed above. Often the most effective arm of treatment will be transfer of the patient to a quieter room with optimal sensory and orienting stimuli on the regular nursing floor.

Some patients who have recovered from the acute effects of delirium will suffer a "stress response syndrome."[28] Considerable emotional distress, bewilderment, and embarrassment may follow what the patient retrospectively regards as an unacceptable or frightening loss of control. Such reactions emphasize the importance of routine follow-up after the acute phase of treatment. Explanation and reassurance are helpful. On the other hand, failure by the patient to acknowledge the occurrence of delirium or the inability to tolerate such loss of control may be a clue to underlying personality disturbance (Murray GB, personal communication, 1983).

CONCLUSION

Despite the psychologic threats faced during their illness and its treatment, most cardiac patients retain psychologic equilibrium. Still, the average patient who has had an MI or awaits cardiac surgery has experienced anxiety and its disquieting effects. Supportive measures as well as anxiolytic medication will assist the majority of patients in overcoming these difficulties. Moreover, the ability to employ denial adaptively may help the patient through in-hospital crises.

In many patients, anxiety will be accompanied by depressed mood, engendered by a sense of loss or helplessness. Here, again, supportive measures are often all that is necessary to assist these patients. However, certain patients will be overwhelmed by their anxiety, and as a result will manifest maladaptive personality traits and defense mechanisms. In other instances, cause and effect may be reversed: premorbid psychiatric illness or personality disorder may precipitate severe anxious and depressive reactions and inappropriate behavior. Confrontation, limit-setting, and appeals for cooperation are often useful in the treatment of such patients.

Delirium is often the end point for those least able to tolerate the rigorous demands of care in the CCU or surgical recovery room. Prolonged confinement, restriction, monotony, and noise - features endemic to the intensive care unit environment - are disorienting and stressful influences, particularly in the aged and in those with underlying organic, metabolic, or toxic disturbances. Correction of these abnormalities may reverse delirium, but more often than not a specific abnormality cannot be identified, and neuroleptic medication is required for effective treatment.

In general, no one treatment approach to the hospitalized cardiac patient is sufficient. Patients usually present a constellation of psychiatric problems and symptoms requiring assessment of a multitude of potential psychologic as well as medical determinants. The skilled intensive care unit nurse and medical/surgical team are competent to treat most of these, but when difficult problems persist, psychiatric intervention is required.

REFERENCES

1. Jenkins CD, Stanton B, Savageau JA, Denlinger P, Klein MD: Coronary artery bypass surgery: Physical, psychological, social, and economic outcomes six months later. *JAMA* 1983;250:782-788.
2. Lloyd GG, Cawley RH: Distress or illness? A study of psychological symptoms after myocardial infarction. *Br J Psychiatry* 1983;142:120-125.
3. Cay EL, Vetter N, Philip AE: Psychological status during recovery from an acute heart attack. *J Psychosom Res* 1972;16:437-447.
4. Dominion J, Dobson M: Study of patients' psychological attitudes to a coronary care unit. *Br Med J* 1969;4:795-798.
5. Hackett TP, Cassem NH, Wishnie HA: The coronary-care unit: An appraisal of its psychological hazards. *N Engl J Med* 1968;279:1365-1370.

6. Cassem NH: Psychiatric problems in patients with acute myocardial infarction, in Karliner JS, Gregoratos G (eds): *Coronary Care.* New York, Churchill Livingstone, 1981:829-846.
7. Lynch JJ: The effect of human contact on cardiac rhythm in coronary care patients. *J Nerv Ment Dis* 1974; 158:88-99.
8. Hackett TP, Cassem NH: Psychological intervention in acute myocardial infarction, Gentry WD, Williams RB (eds): *Psychological Aspects of Myocardial Infarction and Coronary Care.* St. Louis, C. V. Mosby, 1979:149-161.
9. Hoffman M, Donckers S, Hauser M: The effect of nursing intervention on stress factors perceived by patients in a coronary care unit. *Heart Lung* 1978;7:804-809.
10. Froese A, Hackett TP, Cassem NH, Silverberg EL: Trajectories of anxiety and depression in denying and non-denying acute MI patients during hospitalization. *J Psychosom Res* 1974;18:413-420.
11. Groves JE: Taking care of the hateful patient. *N Engl J Med* 1978;298:883-887.
12. Parker DL, Hodge JR: Delirium in a coronary care unit. *JAMA* 1967;201:702-703.
13. Gentry WD: Type A/B responses to acute MI. *Heart Lung* 1981;10:1101-1105.
14. Baile WF, Brinker JA, Wachspress JD, Engel BT: Signouts against medical advice from a coronary care unit. *J Behav Med* 1979;2:85-92.
15. Dubin WR, Field HL, Gastfriend DR: Postcardiotomy delirium: A critical review. *J Thorac Cardiovasc Surg* 1979;77:586-594.
16. McKegney FP: The intensive care syndrome. *Conn Med* 1966;30:633-636.
17. Kornfeld DS, Heller SS, Frank KA, Edie RN, Barsal J: Delirium after coronary artery bypass surgery. *J Thorac Cardiovasc Surg* 1978;76:93-96.
18. Razin AM: Psychosocial intervention in CAD: A review. *Psychosom Med* 1982;44:363-387.
19. Thompson TL, Thompson WL: Treating postoperative delirium. *Drug Ther* 1983;13:30-40.
20. Cassem NH, Sos J: Intravenous use of haloperidol for acute delirium in intensive care settings. *Drug Ther* 1980; 10:103-106.
21. Cassano GB, Maggini C, Guazzelli M: Nocturnal angina and sleep. *Prog Neuropsychopharmacol Biol Psychiatry* 1981;5:99-104.

22. Klein RF, Kliner VA, Zipes DP, Troyer WG, Wallace AG: Transfer from a coronary care unit. *Arch Intern Med* 1968;122:104-108.
23. Merwin BS, Abram HS: Psychological response to coronary artery bypass. *South Med J* 1977;70:153-155.
24. Surman OS, Hackett TP, Silverberg EL, Behrendt DM: Usefulness of psychiatric intervention in patients undergoing cardiac surgery. *Arch Gen Psychiatry* 1974;30:830-835.
25. Willner AE, Rabiner CJ, Wisoff BG, Fishman J, Rosen B, Harstein M, Klein DF: Analogy tests and psychopathology at follow-up after open heart surgery. *Biol Psychiatry* 1976;11:687-696.
26. Nadelson T: The psychiatrist in the surgical intensive care unit. *Arch Surg* 1976;111:113-117.
27. Tune LE, Holland A, Folstein MF, Damlouji NF, Gardner TJ, Coyle JT: Association of postoperative delirium with raised serum levels of anticholinergic drugs. *Lancet* 1981;2:651-653.
28. MacKenzie TB, Popkin MK: Stress response syndrome occurring after delirium. *Am J Psychiatry* 1980;137:1433-1435.

6

Biobehavioral Treatment Approaches for Cardiovascular Disorders*

Margaret A. Chesney and Marcia M. Ward

There is extensive clinical and research literature that links psychologic stress with cardiovascular diseases, and in particular to hypertension,[1] coronary heart disease,[2] cardiac arrhythmias,[3] and sudden death.[4] Research has shown that certain emotional and behavioral responses to environmental stress are factors in the development and the progression of cardiovascular disease. The specific nature of the impact of stress on the patient, including the manner in which stress interacts with environmental factors and individual characteristics to increase risk, remains elusive. As a result, efforts to minimize cardiovascular risk using biobehavioral treatments have typically emphasized stress management techniques, which are designed to decrease levels of general arousal.

Relaxation and biofeedback training were the first stress management techniques applied in an effort to reduce cardiovascular risk. Recently, expanded biobehavioral strategies have been developed and applied in the treatment and prevention of cardiovascular disease. One direction this expansion has taken has been the training of patients in the application of relaxation skills to stressful situations in the natural environment. Another major direction that stress management has followed emphasizes modification of the patient's cognitive appraisal of, and response to, situations as either challenging or stressful.

---

*Supported by Grant HL24416 from the National Heart, Lung, and Blood Institute.

Descriptions of the four leading stress management strategies - relaxation, biofeedback, anxiety management training, and anger management training - will outline the primary steps involved when used as therapy for patients with cardiovascular disease.

RELAXATION

There is a growing literature suggesting that relaxation techniques (e.g., progressive muscle relaxation, relaxation responses, meditation practices) may be effective in controlling cardiovascular responses to stress and in so doing, may reduce cardiovascular risk. The majority of studies examining the efficacy of relaxation for cardiovascular risk reduction focuses on hypertension. Several reviews[5-8] conclude that training and continued practice of various relaxation techniques may successfully lower blood pressure in those patients with essential hypertension, although comparative studies suggest that medical treatment may be superior for patients with established hypertension.

MUSCLE RELAXATION

Progressive muscle relaxation (PMR) was originated by Edmund Jacobson[9] as a means of assisting patients to achieve conscious control over skeletal muscles, in order to reduce anxiety, tension, and blood pressure. The PMR program he pioneered focused on training patients how to tense and then to relax separate skeletal muscle groups (e.g., left forearm), progressing through the body with a training session devoted to each muscle group. However, the extensive training time was a major obstacle to the widespread use of Jacobson's procedure. After 1958, however, when Wolpe[10] reported that an abbreviated form of PMR was effective in treating anxiety-related disorders, relaxation technique began to achieve widespread use. This shortened version, with minor variations, is the most extensively studied and applied form of relaxation training today.

Research on the components of relaxation treatment necessary for effective treatment has identified four important factors: (a) achievement of muscular relaxation, (b) control of mental activity by focusing attention on the exercise or on relaxing imagery, (c) regular practice, and (d) the patient's expectation of success in achieving the treatment goal. A typical PMR treatment program, including these four components, might begin with an introductory session with the patient, explaining the rationale and providing an overview of the biobehavioral intervention in order to enhance expectancy. In the following sessions, subjects are trained in a series of four exercises. The basic component of the first three exercises follows Jacobson's original tense-relax method, in which patients, reclining in a quiet relaxed setting, are instructed by a therapist to tense (for 5 to 7 seconds) and then to relax certain specific muscle groups, focusing on the difference between sensations associated with tension and those associated with relaxation. This method brings into play important muscle relaxation and mental focusing components as noted previously. Shown in Table 1, the first three exercises in this typical program involve taking successively fewer muscle groups through the tense and relax method.

Once patients have demonstrated a proficiency in the first three exercises, they are instructed to count backward from 10 to 1 while simultaneously maintaining deep

TABLE 1: TYPICAL PROGRESSIVE MUSCLE RELAXATION EXERCISE SEQUENCE

First Exercise*	Second Exercise	Third Exercise
Right hand and forearm	Right arm and hand	Right and left arms and hands
Left hand and forearm	Left arm and hand	Face, head, and neck
Biceps	Face	Shoulders, upper back, chest, and stomach
Forehead	Head and neck	Left and right legs
Eyes	Shoulders and upper back	
Head and neck	Chest and stomach	
Shoulders and upper back	Buttocks and thighs	
Chest	Calves	
Stomach		
Buttocks		
Thighs		
Calves		

*The patient is instructed to tense and, after holding the tension for 5 to 7 seconds, then relax each muscle group in each exercise sequence.

diaphragmatic breathing. With each number, they are instructed to take a deep breath, review the status of their muscle groups, and identify any pre-existing tension. Then, as they exhale, they are instructed to release the tension and relax the muscle group.

These four exercises are taught in sequence, with two 45-50-minute sessions devoted to each exercise. As the patient advances through the training sequence, the time required to achieve tension-reduction shortens. Thus, the briefer relaxation exercises (i.e., three and four) are repeated during the session as time permits. Patients are instructed to practice the most recently learned relaxation exercise on a daily or near-daily basis. To aid in the practice, patients are frequently given audiotapes of the appropriate exercise. Patients are typically asked to keep a diary noting their home practice sessions to be reviewed by the therapist.

RELAXATION RESPONSE

Simpler approaches to relaxation have also been purported to reduce cardiovascular arousal and lower blood pressure in some patients with essential hypertension.[6] These approaches include transcendental meditation, yoga, hypnosis, and autogenic training.[8] Benson[11] identified four criteria common to these techniques: mental focusing on a constant mental stimulus, a passive attitude without concern about performance, decreased muscle focus, and a quiet setting. Benson argues that when these four requirements are met, the same relaxation response is elicited as is brought about by the more "cultic" techniques such as meditation and yoga. To elicit the relaxation response, Benson instructed patients to sit quietly with their eyes closed and relax all their muscles, starting with their feet and progressing to their face. The instructor tells the patients to breathe through their nose, focus on their breathing, and silently repeat the number "one" as they exhale. They are instructed to do this for 20 minutes, once or twice each day, and are told to not worry about their performance or whether or not they are successful. To the contrary, they are asked to maintain a passive attitude, ignoring distractions and permitting the relaxation response to proceed on its own throughout the exercise. Benson and colleagues[12] have reported clinical case studies indicating that the relaxation response may be an effective strategy for the reduction of blood pressure in motivated patients, thereby reducing the occurrence of cardiac arrhythmias.

BIOFEEDBACK

Biofeedback involves the use of noninvasive instrumentation as a means of providing continuous information to a patient about specific physiologic processes controlled by the autonomic nervous system. Historically, physiologic responses were believed to be controlled by the autonomic nervous system. However, research in animals has demonstrated that numerous responses mediated by the autonomic nervous system can be brought under the animal's control using operant conditioning. These procedures were attempted in humans and their success led to the clinical application of these techniques to psychophysiologic disorders.

In the clinic, biofeedback training takes place in a controlled environment where the patient can focus attention on one specific response modality at a time. As the physiologic response is measured, continuous feedback of the level of physiologic activity is provided. In addition, reinforcers (e.g., lights, tones, or colored bars on a video terminal) are presented to the patient whenever the physiologic activity changes in the desired direction. The individual learns how to control physiologic activity by using feedback and the reinforcers to successively approximate and ultimately produce the correct response. Once some degree of control has been achieved, progressively larger changes in the desired direction are required before reinforcement is given. This shaping procedure facilitates learning and increases the patient's degree of control over the physiologic response system. It is through the application of these operant conditioning techniques that the individual learns to control physiologic activity and to eliminate a maladaptive response pattern that may be producing a patient's psychophysiologic disorder.[13]

The list of autonomic nervous system responses that can be modified using these techniques includes: heart rate, blood pressure, skin temperature, electrodermal activity, muscle activity, stomach motility, and electroencephalographic rhythms. The list of cardiovascular disorders that can be treated with biofeedback includes: hypertension, cardiac arrhythmias, and vascular or migraine headaches.

BIOFEEDBACK TREATMENTS FOR HYPERTENSION

Biofeedback treatments for hypertension have developed in two major directions. The first method of treatment involves feedback of blood pressure levels to teach the patient how to directly control blood pressure. However, because of the difficulty in providing continuous measurements of blood pressure level, a second direction involving biofeedback of other physiologic parameters is more often employed in the clinic. For this approach, continuous measurements of noncardiovascular indexes, for example, electrodermal activity or muscle activity, are provided as a reference guide to aid the individual in learning the techniques of general relaxation and stress management. Biofeedback techniques and the results of research employing the use of biofeedback as a means of controlling hypertension are reviewed as follows.

Blood Pressure Feedback. The blood pressure biofeedback device most often used is the "constant cuff" developed by Tursky and associates.[14] It consists of a sphygmomanometer with a microphone built into the cuff. To obtain beat-by-beat measurements of relative blood pressure, the cuff is inflated to the level where Korotkoff sounds are heard 50% of the time. This level is equivalent to the median systolic blood pressure level (e.g., 140 mm Hg) at that moment. The patient is given binary feedback on whether the Korotkoff sound is present or not. When systolic blood pressure decreases below the pressure in the cuff (e.g., 138 mm Hg), no Korotkoff sounds are heard. When systolic blood pressure increases above the pressure in the cuff (e.g., 142 mm Hg), Korotkoff sounds become audible. The patient is instructed to "keep the Korotkoff sounds off." During training sessions, the relative absence of Korotkoff sounds indicates a decrease in systolic blood pressure and signifies success. Conversely, the predominance of Korotkoff sounds indicates an increase in systolic blood pressure and means failure. Thus, patients are provided with nearly continuous information about their relative systolic blood pressure during feedback periods, or trials, that last approximately 50 seconds.

Once patients are able to maintain their blood pressure at a given level for several trials, the cuff pressure can be set lower and the patient may be given the same instructions, for example, "turn off" the Korotkoff sounds. Used in this manner, biofeedback can improve or "shape" the patient's blood pressure control. This "constant cuff" system has been used in a number of studies regarding blood pressure biofeedback in normotensives by Shapiro and colleagues[15,16] with noted success. However, there is no constant cuff device commercially available, which limits its clinical usage.

A readily available and easy technique for providing feedback of blood pressure levels involves the use of standard blood pressure cuffs in order to measure absolute blood pressure levels on a periodic basis. To increase the frequency of readings without added discomfort and risk of venous pooling, a cuff often is placed on each arm and the cuffs are inflated alternately. This system is inexpensive, but it only provides feedback of blood pressure levels once every 30 seconds.

A measure related to blood pressure level is the pulse-wave velocity or pulse transit time, for example, the transit time of the pulse signal from the heart to the radial artery in the wrist. This provides a comfortable and continuous reading using commercially available devices. Initial studies have reported that learned control of pulse transit time can help to lower blood pressure.[17,18] However, there is some dispute over how well pulse-wave velocity is correlated with blood pressure.[19-21]

Biofeedback-Assisted Relaxation. Biofeedback has also been used to facilitate relaxation, and thus to indirectly lower blood pressure levels. Feedback of sympathetically innervated responses such as electrodermal activity and muscle activity is provided and used to teach individuals control of sympathetic nervous system activity while they are learning relaxation. This approach has been used successfully in a number of studies of hypertension, including several by Patel and colleagues.[22-24]

Effectiveness of Biofeedback Training for Hypertension. The effectiveness of various types of biofeedback training for reducing blood pressure has been previously evaluated and reviewed.[25-27] Taylor[27] reported that biofeedback-assisted relaxation leads to reduction in systolic blood pressure of 8 to 28 mm Hg and reduction in diastolic blood pressure of 8 to 19 mm Hg. However, critical reviews of blood pressure biofeedback technique conclude that there is no advantage of the biofeedback method when compared with relaxation training. For example, Agras and Jacob[25] concluded that "feedback of blood pressure has no greater clinical effect than relaxation therapy, thus the extra investment in blood pressure feedback equipment would seem unwarranted unless more sophisticated and powerful methods are developed."

BIOFEEDBACK TREATMENT FOR CARDIAC ARRHYTHMIAS

Biofeedback has been reported as a treatment for cardiac arrhythmias in a handful of case reports and small population studies. Feuerstein and Ward[3] reviewed these studies separately for biofeedback treatments of premature ventricular contractions (PVCs) and tachycardia.

Heart rate feedback has been used in the treatment of PVCs and has resulted in the elimination or reduction in frequency of PVCs in approximately 50% of reported case studies. The most effective biofeedback treatment for PVCs involves training the patient first to alternately accelerate and decelerate heart rate and then to maintain heart rate within a fixed range. Training in heart rate deceleration has been the most common therapeutic strategy for the biobehavioral treatment of tachycardia. This approach may be facilitated by teaching heart rate control in the presence of stressful stimuli.

Although the literature contains reports of successful treatment of cardiac arrhythmias with biobehavioral techniques, the number of cases treated is very limited. If biobehavioral approaches are to be attempted, Feuerstein and Ward[3] suggest the initial use of muscle relaxation training or relaxation response[12] in an effort to decrease general sympathetic arousal. If necessary, this training could be followed by heart rate biofeedback to reduce cardiac arrhythmic activity and training to reduce stress-induced arrhythmias in the presence of specific stressors.

ANXIETY MANAGEMENT TRAINING

Anxiety management training (AMT) was developed in 1971 by Suinn and Richardson[28] as a conditioning procedure designed to reduce anxiety reactions. It was designed to be a brief therapy or intervention that would provide patients with a stress management skill easily applied to any tension-producing situation.

In practice, AMT is usually taught in three stages. The first step is to teach relaxation techniques such as those discussed previously. Once the patients have learned to attain a relaxed state, they are instructed to imagine and visualize a situation that produces an anxiety reaction. Patients are instructed to recognize the physical sensations of anxiety and then to put the situation or scene out of their minds and to shift to implementation of their relaxation skills until a deep level of relaxation is attained. This procedure is repeated numerous times using a variety of anxiety-producing scenes until patients learn or are "conditioned" to shift "automatically" to a relaxed state when anxiety occurs.

Suinn[29] has developed a version of AMT specifically for use in cardiac rehabilitation programs for controlling responsivity to stress in Type A individuals (see also Chapter 7). This technique is called cardiac stress management training and supplements AMT with an emphasis on controlling the stress resulting from time-urgent events. Suinn and Bloom[30] remark that patients believed that their levels of anxiety and Type A behavior were reduced after training; however, no reductions in blood pressure, cholesterol, or triglyceride levels were attained. Jenni and Wollersheim[31] also reported that self-perceived levels of Type A behavior and anxiety were reduced in normotensives after AMT training.

Recently, AMT has been applied to hypertension with encouraging results.[32,33] In one study,[33] 18 hypertensive patients showed significant reductions in both systolic and diastolic blood pressure immediately post-treatment, with a further reduction after a 6-week follow-up. Moreover, AMT decreased the patients' systolic and diastolic blood pressure responses to a cognitively challenging task, indicating the efficacy of the treatment for stress management. Though research on the application of AMT to hypertension is limited, the results are promising, particularly in terms of blood pressure control during actual stress, and will undoubtedly encourage further clinical research of this technique.

ANGER MANAGEMENT TRAINING

Recently, anger and hostility have been implicated in the pathogenesis of cardiovascular disease. Hostility as an attitudinal set involving suspiciousness and mistrust may be the major "coronary-prone" component of the Type A behavior pattern.[34] Hostility has also been shown to be related to the extent of coronary artery disease as assessed by angiography and to predict a 20-year risk of death from all causes, including coronary heart disease.[35] Although the manner in which this individual characteristic leads to increased cardiovascular disease has yet to be elucidated, there is considerable speculation that hostile individuals perceive more situations as challenging and respond to those challenges with commensurate levels of sympathetic nervous system arousal. In response to a laboratory task involving a modest level of challenge, Type A individuals who scored high on a measure of hostility showed greater cardiovascular responses than did Type A persons who scored low in hostility.[36]

There is also evidence that anger or hostility is related to elevated blood pressure. In particular, there are a number of studies suggesting that hypertensive patients possess increased levels of anger of hostility when compared with normotensive subjects. For example, Harburg and colleagues[37,38] have shown that a response to provocation with anger is associated with elevated blood pressure in people regardless of race or sex. In a prospective study, Barefoot and associates[39] noted that 13 of 20 individuals who showed high levels of hostility during medical school were later found to be hypertensive at a 25-year follow-up. In a review of three independent studies, Julius[40] pointed out that those "patients with high-renin, mild hypertension demonstrated suppressed hostility, and had hostile feelings of suspicion and resentment, were irritable, and were given to verbal aggressive actions." These findings suggest that a promising target for stress management and cardiovascular disease risk reduction may be the hostile cognitive style or attitudinal set and the emotional state of anger.[41]

Anger management training offers an approach that is well suited for cardiovascular patients. It has been found to lower blood pressure responses in reaction to anger-provoking situations in normotensive young adults,[42] as well as in psychiatric outpatients,[43] and has also proved to be an effective adjunct in stress management training for both hypertensive patients and cardiac rehabilitation patients after myocardial infarction and coronary artery bypass (graft) surgery.

There are three treatment phases in anger management training. In the first, cognitive preparation, the focus is on the individual's perception or appraisal of a situation as anger arousing. Events are not characterized as anger provoking per se, but obtain this quality based upon their interpretation by the individual. The patient is educated about anger arousal and its determinants and is taught to self-monitor (i.e., observe and record behavioral responses to situations in a diary). Self-monitoring is used to identify circumstances that elicit or trigger anger and to use this information as a means of discriminating between adaptive and maladaptive occurrences of anger. At the end of this first treatment phase, patients are introduced to anger management techniques as valuable coping strategies for helping patients to effectively handle stress and conflict situations.

The second phase of treatment, skill acquisition, involves recognition of the determinants and manifestation of anger, discussion of alternative coping strategies, modeling of these techniques by the therapist, and practice by the patient. Novaco[41] notes that when a hostile patient appraises a situation as a personal insult or challenge, this appraisal must be questioned. Learning not to "take things personally" and instead to maintain a task orientation, rather than a personal orientation, becomes a key focus of the treatment. Another primary emphasis addresses the fact that anger can result from unreasonably high expectations of oneself and others - the person learns to re-adjust these expectations to more realistic levels. In most cases, patients' self-monitoring reveals a pattern of becoming angry in some predictable, routine circumstances. For these instances, training includes "self-instruction," for example, the patients are trained to replace their previously angry appraisals and thoughts about situations with ones that are more adaptive and effective. Relaxation training also is included in the skill acquisition phase. This approach instills in patients the expectation that they can achieve mastery over stressful situations and internal states. Moreover, relaxation training teaches patients a strategy that they can use to delay their typically quick responses to provocation. Such a delay is critical and permits patients to weigh alternative appraisals of and various coping strategies for stressful situations. Another skill included in this treatment phase is assertiveness training.[44] Here, patients are taught nonaggressive communication, as well as how to express a negative viewpoint or sentiment in a nonantagonistic and inoffensive manner.

The third phase of anger management training is application training. The therapist supervises the patient's practice of newly acquired skills in predetermined provocative situations. These situations are often arranged in a hierarchical order and imagery is used to simulate the situations in sequence, thereby evoking the application of newly acquired skills to be used in a manner similar to AMT. Following rehearsal of imagery, patients practice their skills in role-playing situations with therapists and then apply their skills to real situations.

SUMMARY

The four stress management strategies outlined in this chapter reflect the range of biobehavioral approaches to cardiovascular risk reduction. At one end of the spectrum is relaxation training, a well-researched modality that serves as the foundation for other approaches. At the opposite end of the spectrum is anger management training, a newcomer to the biobehavioral repertoire, developed in response to the literature implicating anger and hostility in cardiovascular disease. The rationale for these treatments relies on a presumed association linking emotional and behavioral responses to stress with the development and progression of cardiovascular disease. To the extent that the mechanisms and dynamics underlying this association have not been determined, the active therapeutic components of biobehavioral treatments remain elusive. These active components may include not only such treatment variables as relaxation skills acquisition, but also such nonspecific treatment effects as expectancy, for example, the patient's beliefs regarding the efficacy of the treatment strategy.

Stress management techniques have not yet been evaluated in clinical trials with cardiovascular disease end points. Certainly, one primary objective of such future trials will be to identify the characteristics of patients who are particularly responsive to specific biobehavioral stress management strategies. In the absence of these data, clinical experience suggests that relaxation, either alone or in combination with biofeedback or AMT, is effective in reducing the self-reporting of stress and arousal by patients who experience somatic tension and mental or cognitive tension. When the patient perceives stressful situations as anger provoking, biobehavioral treatments such as anger management training may be more beneficial. In fact, recent data collected in our laboratory suggest that relaxation was not particularly effective in the lowering of blood pressure among hypertensive patients scoring high on anger arousal, but instead that hypertensive patients scoring low on anger arousal showed decreased blood pressure levels following relaxation and biofeedback training.

The treatment effects observed with biobehavioral techniques, though statistically significant when compared with untreated controls, are modest in comparison with the effects of standard medical regimens, for example, antihypertensive medication. Consequently, these techniques are usually recommended as an adjunct to medical management, or as is the case in hypertension, they are advocated as a preliminary treatment step for patients with diastolic blood pressures between 90 and 95 mm Hg.

On the positive side, the stress management strategies discussed here appeal to patients interested in managing their own stress. These approaches not only make sense intuitively, but they introduce patients to skills in physiologic arousal reduction that can be initiated at will. While we await the results of necessary clinical trials, these strategies will continue to have a place in the treatment of the patient with cardiovascular disease simply because they do not appear to result in negative side effects. Moreover, they enhance the patient's perception of self-control over stress and may reduce cardiovascular arousal to stress.

REFERENCES

1. Obrist PA, Langer AW, Grignolo A, Light KC, Hastrup JL, McCubbin JA, Koepke JP, Pollock MH: Behavioral-cardiac interactions in hypertension, in Krantz DS, Baum A, Singer JE (eds): *Cardiovascular Disorders and Behavior.* Hillsdale, NJ, Lawrence Erlbaum, 1983.
2. Rosenman RH, Chesney MA: Stress, type A behavior, and coronary disease, in Goldberger L, Breznitz S (eds): *Handbook of Stress: Theoretical and Clinical Aspects.* New York, Macmillan, 1982:547-565.
3. Feuerstein M, Ward MM: Psychological treatment of cardiac arrhythmias, in Ferguson JM, Taylor CB (eds): *The Comprehensive Handbook of Behavioral Medicine.* New York, Spectrum Publications, 1980.
4. Verrier RL, DeSilva RA, Lown B: Psychological factors in cardiac arrhythmias and sudden death, in Krantz

DS, Baum A, Singer J (eds): *Cardiovascular Disorders and Behavior.* Hillsdale, NJ, Lawrence Erlbaum, 1983.
5. Shapiro D, Goldstein IB: Biobehavioral perspectives on hypertension. *J Consult Clin Psychol* 1982;50:841-858.
6. Jacob RG, Kraemer HC, Agras WS: Relaxation therapy in the treatment of hypertension. *Arch Gen Psychol* 1977;34:1417-1427.
7. Shapiro AP, Jacob RG: Nonpharmacologic approaches to the treatment of hypertension. *Annu Rev Pub Health* 1983;4:285-310.
8. Frumkin K, Nathan RJ, Prout MF, Cohen MC: Nonpharmacologic control of essential hypertension in man: A critical review of the experimental literature. *Psychosom Med* 1978;40:294-320.
9. Jacobson E: Use of relaxation in hypertensive states. *NY State J Med* 1920;111:419-422.
10. Wolpe J: *Psychotherapy by Reciprocal Inhibition.* Stanford, Stanford University Press, 1958.
11. Benson H: Systemic hypertension and the relaxation response. *N Engl J Med* 1977;296:1152-1156.
12. Benson H, Alexander S, Feldman CL: Decreased premature ventricular contractions through use of the relaxation response in patients with stable ischaemic heart disease. *Lancet* 1975;2:380-382.
13. Shapiro D, Surwit RS: Biofeedback, in Pomerleau OF, Brady JP (eds): *Behavioral Medicine: Theory and Practice.* Baltimore, Williams and Wilkins, 1979:45-74.
14. Tursky B, Shapiro D, Schwartz GE: Automated constant cuff-pressure system to measure average systolic and diastolic blood pressure in man. *IEEE Trans Biomed Eng* 1972;19:271-276.
15. Shapiro D, Tursky B, Schwartz GE: Differentiation of heart rate and systolic blood pressure in man by operant conditioning. *Psychosom Med* 1970;32:417-423.
16. Shapiro D, Schwartz GE, Tursky B: Control of diastolic blood pressure in man by feedback and reinforcement. *Psychophysiology* 1972;9:296-304.
17. Steptoe A: Blood pressure control with pulse-wave velocity feedback: Methods of analysis and training, in Beatty J, Legewie H (eds): *Biofeedback and Behavior.* New York, Plenum, 1977:355-368.
18. Steptoe A, Johnston D: The control of blood pressure using pulse-wave velocity feedback. *J Psychosom Res* 1976;20:417-424.
19. Allen RA, Schneider JA, Davidson DM, Winchester MA, Taylor CB: The covariation of blood pressure and

pulse transit time in hypertensive patients. *Psychophysiology* 1981;18:301-306.
20. Lane JD, Greenstadt L, Shapiro D, Rubenstein E: Pulse transit time and blood pressure: An intensive analysis. *Psychophysiology* 1983;20:45-49.
21. Newlin DB: Relationships of pulse transmission times to pre-ejection period and blood pressure. *Psychophysiology* 1981;18:316-321.
22. Patel CH: Yoga and biofeedback in the management of hypertension. *Lancet* 1973;2:1053-1055.
23. Patel CH, North WRS: Randomized control trial of yoga and biofeedback in management of hypertension. *Lancet* 1975;2:93-95.
24. Patel CH: Biofeedback-aided relaxation and meditation in the management of hypertension. *Biofeedback Self Regul* 1977;2:1-41.
25. Agras S, Jacob R: Hypertension, in Pomerleau OF, Brady JP (eds): *Behavioral Medicine: Theory and Practice.* Baltimore, Williams and Wilkins, 1979:205-232.
26. Shapiro AP, Schwartz GE, Ferguson DCE, Redmond DP, Weiss SM: Behavioral methods in the treatment of hypertension. *Ann Intern Med* 1977;86:626-636.
27. Taylor CB: Behavioral approaches to hypertension, in Ferguson JM, Taylor CB (eds): *The Comprehensive Handbook of Behavioral Medicine: I.* New York, Spectrum Publications, 1980:55-88.
28. Suinn RM, Richardson F: Anxiety management training: A nonspecific behavior therapy program for anxiety control. *Behav Ther* 1971;2:498-510.
29. Suinn RM: Behavior therapy for cardiac patients. *Behav Ther* 1974;5:569-571.
30. Suinn RM, Bloom LJ: Anxiety management training for pattern A behavior. *J Behav Med* 1978;1:25-35.
31. Jenni MA, Wollersheim JP: Cognitive therapy, stress management training, and the type A behavior pattern. *Cognitive Therapy Research* 1979;3:61-73.
32. Bloom LJ, Cantrell B: Anxiety management training for essential hypertension in pregnancy. *Behav Ther* 1978; 9:377-382.
33. Jorgensen RS, Houston BK, Zurawski RM: Anxiety management training in the treatment of essential hypertension. *Behav Res Ther* 1981;19:467-474.
34. Rosenman RH: Health consequences of anger and implications for treatment, in Chesney MA, Rosenman RH (eds): *Anger and Hostility in Cardiovascular and Behavioral Disorders.* New York, McGraw-Hill, 1985.

35. Williams RB, Barefoot JC, Shekelle RB: The health consequences of hostility, in Chesney MA, Rosenman RH (eds): *Anger and Hostility in Cardiovascular and Behavioral Disorders.* New York, McGraw-Hill, 1985.
36. Dembroski TM, MacDougall JM, Shields JL, Petitto J, Lushene R: Components of the type A coronary-prone behavior pattern and cardiovascular responses to psychomotor challenge. *J Behav Med* 1978;1:159-176.
37. Gentry WD, Chesney AP, Gary HE, Hall RP, Harburg E: Habitual anger-coping styles: I. Effect on mean blood pressure and risk for essential hypertension. *Psychosom Med* 1982;44:195-202.
38. Harburg E, Erfurt JC, Hauenstein LS, Chape C, Schull WJ, Schork MA: Socio-ecological stress, suppressed hostility, skin color, and black-white male blood pressure: Detroit. *Psychosom Med* 1973;35:276-296.
39. Barefoot JC, Dahlstrom WG, Williams RB: Hostility, CHD incidence, and total mortality: A 25-year follow-up study of 255 physicians. *Psychosom Med* 1983;45:59-63.
40. Julius S: The psychophysiology of borderline hypertension, in Weiner H, Hofer MA, Stunkard AJ (eds): *Brain, Behavior and Disease.* New York, Raven Press, 1981:293-303.
41. Novaco RW: The functions and regulation of the arousal of anger. *Am J Psychiatry* 1976;133:1124-1128.
42. Moon JR, Eisler RM: Anger control: An experimental comparison of three behavioral treatments. *Behav Ther* 1983;14:493-505.
43. Novaco RW: *Anger Control: The Development and Evaluation of an Experimental Treatment.* Lexington, MA, Lexington Press, 1975.
44. Lange AJ, Jakubowski P: *Responsible Assertive Behavior: Cognitive-Behavioral Procedures for Trainers.* Champaign, IL, Research Press, 1976.

7

Altering the Type A Behavior Pattern in Post-Infarction Patients*

Carl E. Thoresen, Meyer Friedman, Lynda H. Powell, James J. Gill, and Diane Ulmer

INTRODUCTION

In the worry and strain of modern life, arterial degeneration is not only very common but develops often at a relatively early age. For this, I believe that the high pressure at which men live and the habit of working the machine to its maximum capacity are responsible rather than excesses in eating and drinking.[1]

Sir William Osler's observation reflects the views of a few other historical figures: how people think, feel, and of course behave in their daily life play a major role in processes directly linked to major diseases. In the case of ischemic heart disease, strong and intimate relationships among emotional factors, health, and disease have long been suspected, dating back at least three centuries to Harvey, Heberden, and Hunter.[2] Despite the astute clinical observations of Osler in the early 1900s that suggested a connection between lifestyle habits and the pathogenesis of heart disease, medical treatment regimens have commonly ignored the area of emotional habits.[3,4] Such avoidance may have been reinforced in part by

---

*The Recurrent Coronary Prevention Project was aided by grants from National Heart, Lung, and Blood Institute (21427), Bank of America, Standard Oil of California, The Kaiser Hospital Foundation, and the Mary Potishman Lard Foundation (Fort Worth, Texas).

shortcomings in the ability of psychologic and psychiatric theory early in this century to explain how human emotions might contribute to vascular disease. In addition, the major emphasis by cardiovascular researchers on electrocardiographic, pharmacologic, and epidemiologic perspectives left little room for considering matters of emotional habits and behavioral patterns.

As they expanded on the psychosocial or personality perspectives of earlier investigators concerned with heart disease,[5,6] Friedman and Rosenman identified a set of behaviors and characteristics that they had repeatedly observed in their post-infarction patients. They began to articulate a constellation of observable behaviors and characteristics, which became known as the Type A behavior pattern (TABP). They noted the ubiquitous sense of impatience and time urgency, the pervasive pattern of extreme competitiveness, and the quickness with which angry behavior and hostile feelings were aroused in these patients. The term "struggle" seemed to capture the essence of these behaviors and characteristics - the incessant struggle to overcome real or imagined obstacles imposed by insufficient time and events, and especially by other persons, many of whom were perceived as acting in competitive, threatening, or challenging ways.

Friedman and Rosenman speculated that this persistent struggle resulted in a chronic state of hyperarousal, both physiologically and behaviorally, manifesting itself in how individuals acted (e.g., rapid, abrupt speech), what they said (e.g., critical comments about others), and, presumably, what they thought (e.g., perceiving others as challenging one's control of situations). Further, they reasoned that underlying these behaviors was a basic, profound feeling of insecurity, a pervasive doubt about the level of one's worthiness in certain contexts, such as the home or work environment. This insecurity seemed to be linked to a fear that the person was not genuinely respected and admired by others. This heightened arousal was associated with a constant striving to seek the symbols of recognition and reward as a way of allaying what appeared to be basic fears of inadequacy and insecurity. Hence, actions such as the TABP served to diminish feelings of insecurity or self-doubt and were strongly reinforcing.

Although Friedman and Rosenman initially recognized that the TABP was a complex behavioral syndrome primarily manifested by particular persons in certain situations, but not in other circumstances (i.e., an interaction between individual and environmental factors), the notion of TABP as a fixed personality trait became popularized.[7] For example, common usage of the term "Type A personality" encouraged a fixed-trait orientation. Indeed, the idea of a Type B personality, routinely defined as the absence of Type A behaviors and characteristics, tended to encourage a highly reductionistic and oversimplified trait conception of TABP.

The consequences of a trait orientation have seriously restricted the quality of conceptual and empirical TABP studies.[8,9] Research has too often categorized people as Type A or B and assumed that all persons so classified could be expected to think, feel, and act in the same ways. A clear need exists to move beyond the global classification of Type A, exploring what components or particular behaviors and characteristics within the clinical syndrome of TABP deserve primary attention.

Despite limitations in conceptualizing and assessing the TABP, the association of this syndrome with coronary heart disease (CHD) has been demonstrated in a variety of laboratory,[10-12] clinical,[13-16] and epidemiologic studies.[17,18] A panel of behavioral and medical scientists convened by the National Heart, Lung, and Blood Institute concluded that substantial evidence exists to support an association between the TABP and CHD.[19] Although studies have demonstrated a predictive relationship between TABP and cardiovascular indexes (and some have provided equivocal results), two major questions still remain about the TABP: Can the pattern be substantially altered and, if so, will such change be associated with significant reductions in indicators of CHD? A major research question for any modifiable CHD risk factor is whether a change in that risk factor will be associated with any evidence of a decrease in incidence of some kind in coronary disease.

ALTERING THE TYPE A BEHAVIOR PATTERN

INTERVENTION STUDIES

Although hundreds of published studies have examined the correlates of TABP, using the characteristics as an independent or moderator variable,[7,20] very few controlled intervention studies have sought to alter the TABP directly.[9,21] Still fewer studies have demonstrated significant changes in meaningful CHD criteria. Unfortunately, investigators have generally failed to realize that the two major measures of TABP - the Structured Interview (SI) and the Jenkins Activity Survey (JAS) - do not measure the same features of the TABP.[22] Correlations between the two measures typically range between .22 and .35, indicating a positive yet weak relationship. The SI yields information on speech stylistics coupled with anger and hostility symptoms (e.g., loud or explosive speech, rapid speech, speech interruptions, surly or condescending tone, and anger not expressed directly) and, to a lesser extent, the degree of pressured drive, competitiveness, and impatience. By contrast, the JAS examines the TABP from a job-involvement perspective, with attention to impatience as well as to hard-driving competitiveness. More importantly for treatment, the JAS asks persons to rate themselves on some dimensions (e.g., work history) that could not be expected to change with treatment. In addition, in completing a questionnaire, one is asked to make personal discriminations about oneself that are difficult to do even under the best of conditions. For example, a subject may not readily admit that he or she chronically experiences pervasively hostile feelings and thoughts or an exaggerated sense of competition about most daily activities. One does not ask a patient, as the sole or even primary basis of diagnosis, if he or she has high blood pressure or an elevated serum cholesterol level. Instead, standardized, objective assays that do not rely on a patient's subjective perceptions are used. Patient perceptions and beliefs can clearly play a role in medical diagnosis, but not as the only or basic source of diagnostic evidence. At present, the SI is the most objective and valid means of assessing changes in TABP. The use of questionnaires can complement, but cannot substitute for, the Structured Interview.

Of 16 TABP intervention studies published or in progress at the time of preparation of this review in early 1985,[9] with one exception, none had used the SI to assess changes in the TABP. Some had used "homemade" questionnaires and others have relied on the JAS. Of those studies reporting significant changes, questions arise as to how much confidence and importance can be placed on those self-reported changes. For example, in one of the better designed treatment studies, Levenkron and co-workers[23] found a statistically significant reduction on the JAS Type A scale for healthy men who had attended eight weekly sessions of insight-oriented psychotherapy or received cognitive-behavior therapy. However, social desirability and strong treatment expectancy factors could have readily directed such persons, who volunteered to receive 2 months of treatment, to self-report at the end of treatment that they now had fewer Type A characteristics. How confident can we be that an average reduction of 6.4 points on a self-report scale signifies an actual reduction in Type A behavior in everyday life? Clearly, if treatment seeks to modify the TABP, then robust objective measures of change are essential, especially if one wishes to argue that such changes are in some way linked to changes in certain physiologic measures.

A number of other problems exist with the few TABP intervention studies reported to date. Chief among them are problems of therapy assessment, treatment methods, and the focus and duration of therapy. Typically, treatments have been offered in 8- to 12-hour sessions spread over 2 or 3 months. Furthermore, most published studies have involved older adolescents or adults in their second or third decade who do not yet evidence cardiovascular symptoms. Very few studies have carefully examined the relationship of reductions in TABP and cardiovascular variables in patients after myocardial infarction.

Table 1 (pages 102-103) presents the focus of treatment for selected studies in terms of four major areas: cognitive, behavioral, physiologic, and environmental. In addition, therapy focus (targets), sample size, and treatment duration (in terms of total weeks and total hours) are presented along with the types of measures used, such as a paper-pencil self-report (S) or a biochemical assay (B). Most studies have employed a short-term intervention focused on selected physiologic variables (e.g., serum cholesterol level or blood pressure). None of the studies, with the exception of the Recurrent Coronary Prevention Project (RCPP), have used a more objective measure of TABP, namely the SI, as the primary means to assess change in TABP. Further, except for the RCPP, other studies have not established a relationship between changes in TABP and change in clinically significant CHD measures.

TABLE 1: TREATMENT FOCUS AND MEASURES OF SELECTED TYPE A BEHAVIOR PATTERN INTERVENTION STUDIES

Study	Treatment Focus				Measures Used to Assess Treatment			
	Cognitive	Behavioral	Physiologic	Environmental	Cognitive	Behavioral	Physiologic	Environmental
Suinn[24] N = 30* Treatment: 2 wk (5 hrs)**		X	X		S		B	
Suinn & Bloom[25] N = 14 Treatment: 3 wk (6 hrs)			X		S,P	P	E,B	
Jenni & Wollersheim[26] N = 42 Treatment: 6 wks (9 hrs)	X		X			P	P,E,B	
Roskies et al[27] N = 33 Treatment: 20 wks (14 hrs)	X		X		S,P	S,P,E	S,P,E,B	

Study	Treatment Focus				Measures Used to Assess Treatment			
	Cognitive	Behavioral	Physiologic	Environmental	Cognitive	Behavioral	Physiologic	Environmental
Levenkron et al[23] $\underline{N}$ = 38 Treatment: 8 wks (12 hrs)		X	X	X	S,P	S,P	S,P,E,B	S
Friedman et al[28-31]* $\underline{N}$ = 1,012* Treatment: 4-1/2 yrs (100 hrs)	X	X	X	X	S,P	S,P,E	S,E,B	S,P

* Subjects were post-infarction patients.
** Total treatment time in parentheses.
S = self-report; P = standardized psychometric instrument; E = external observers; B = biochemical assay; N = number of patients.

RECURRENT CORONARY PREVENTION PROJECT

To provide information on altering the TABP and evidence linking change in the TABP to clinical CHD, a 5-year clinical trial, the Recurrent Coronary Prevention Project (RCPP), was initiated in 1977 with 1,012 patients who had a myocardial infarction. The RCPP sought to determine: (a) if the TABP could be altered and, if so, to what extent; and (b) if the TABP could be altered, would subjects demonstrating such modification be more immune to subsequent cardiac recurrences? Details of the research design, subject characteristics, initial reductions in TABP, and coronary morbidity and mortality for the first 3 years have been reported elsewhere.[28-31] Here, some subject characteristics and treatment results will be briefly presented, with a focus on the treatment program.

SUBJECTS' CHARACTERISTICS

A total of 862 subjects volunteered for treatment and were randomly assigned to either cardiologic counseling or cardiologic counseling plus Type A behavioral counseling. Another 150 subjects who did not volunteer for treatment were drawn from the coronary patient population in the San Francisco and Sacramento areas. These subjects volunteered to serve as nontreatment control subjects (medical examinations and TABP assessments only).

The typical subject at entry was a 53-year-old man, 69 inches tall, 170-179 lbs, married, with at least a high school education. Approximately 8% of the subjects were women ($N = 84$). To qualify, a subject must have suffered a documented acute myocardial infarction at least 6 months earlier, not be currently smoking, and never have been treated for or exhibited signs of diabetes. Roughly one in four had already undergone coronary artery bypass graft surgery, one in five had suffered at least two infarctions prior to entry, two in five suffered from hypertension, one in ten had congestive heart failure, and three in four were former smokers. The mean serum cholesterol level at entry was 259.6 + 48.3 mg/dl. Each subject was administered a participant questionnaire (88 items, five-point multiple choice format) that elicited information about specific Type A habits and reactions in common everyday situations. The questionnaire was completed at entry and yearly thereafter. The participant questionnaire consists of several factors, such as hostility, time urgency, and Type A speech/conversational style. Internal consistency of the participant questionnaire is .92 (Cronbach alpha) with a test-retest correlation of .84 over 4 months.

To substantiate the validity of subjects' self-reports, spouses independently completed a separate 43-item spouse questionnaire annually, assessing their perceptions of spouses' Type A behavior. In addition, co-workers completed a 41-item monitor questionnaire that assessed patients' specific Type A behaviors observable in the work environment. Internal consistency and test-retest correlation data were .87/.86 and .80/.73 for the spouse and monitor questionnaires, respectively.

Given the marked limitations of self-report instruments in assessing TABP, primary reliance for assessing change in the TABP was placed in the Video-Taped Structured Interview (VSI), a revision of the original SI developed to categorize subjects as Type A or B in the Western Collaborative Group Study.[32] The VSI has been fully described elsewhere.[28,31] Briefly, a 15-minute interview composed of 28 questions was conducted by an interviewer using an empathic style who was not aware of the subject's treatment status. A total of 38 indicators of speech stylistics, motor behavior, and attitudes were sought and then rated. If an indicator was observed, it was then rated on a scale of 1-3 for intensity. Examples of indicators include hostile or tense facial expression, fast and jerky movements, interruption of the interviewer, and re-experience of anger about past events. All subjects completed a VSI at entry and again after 36 months. Internal consistency of VSI was .74 with test-retest correlation of .76. The percent agreement on 135 subjects rated on both the VSI and the SI used in the Western Collaborative Group Study was 83.6.

TREATMENT PROCEDURES

Treatment concerning the Type A behavioral group counseling and the cardiologic group counseling has been previously described.[29] Currently, a monograph describing treatment is being prepared by the first author and others. However, we will briefly illustrate some examples of Type A behavioral counseling and present some clinical conjectures based on conducting these groups with post-infarction patients.

Cardiologic Group Counseling. In effect, this treatment served as a competing treatment group to control for the possible effects of volunteering for experimental treatment on recurrence rates and TABP. This condition also controlled for factors such as meeting regularly in small groups with a professional leader (cardiologist), receiving advice and information concerning cardiovascular disease and cardiology, and repeatedly completing a variety of assessment measures. Subjects in groups of 12 attended 90-minute cardiologist-led group sessions, biweekly for the first 3 months, monthly for 3 months, and bimonthly for the remainder of the study. A total of 22 such groups focused on the following topics using lectures and discussions, slide presentations, and group discussion procedures: (a) pathogenesis of myocardial infarction, (b) alteration of standard coronary risk factors (e.g., hypertension, hypercholesterolemia, etc.) except TABP, (c) current advances in surgical and drug management of CHD, (d) avoidance of certain daily activities suspected of possibly precipitating recurrent cardiac events (e.g., excessive sudden physical exertion, excessive caffeine or alcohol intake, fatty meals), and (e) compliance with dietary, drug, and exercise prescriptions written by the subject's own personal physician. Cardiologic counseling served as a supplement to medical care already provided by each subject's own physician. In addition, these groups were led every 3 months by a psychologist or psychiatrist who advised them on problems of anxiety, depression, and phobias. However, attention was not given to the TABP (i.e., how to alter selected Type A behaviors and characteristics), or to the topic of chronic stress in general. Otherwise, the cardiologic counseling treatment provided a full spectrum of cardiologic information, advice, and support.

Type A Behavioral/Cardiologic Group Counseling. Subjects received the cardiologic counseling plus behavioral counseling designed to help subjects recognize their own TABP and to modify it. A total of 60 groups of approximately 10 per group met weekly for 2 months, semimonthly for 4 months, and monthly thereafter. Clearly, the major thrust of this treatment was to modify Type A behavior. To do so, an expanded cognitive social learning model was used. This model views ongoing human experience as a function of the interplay of four major factors: cognitive, physiologic, behavioral, and environmental.[33] The key Type A theme of chronic struggle was presented to subjects in terms of these four reciprocal factors. Thus, subjects discussed specific short-term behavioral goals associated with these four areas. For example, in terms of behavioral factors, subjects focused on such actions as speaking more slowly, interrupting others less often, and being more patient and relaxed while waiting in lines or driving cars. Environmentally, attention was given to the establishment of a time and place at home for relaxation practice (at least 20 minutes daily), contracting with spouse or work supervisor about reasonable deadlines, and driving in the right or slower traffic lane. Physiologically, each subject was strongly encouraged to avoid eating heavy meals rich in fats, to practice relaxation skills daily, to take all medications as directed, and to use various relaxation methods (e.g., deep breathing or autogenic phrases) during the day to maintain lower physiologic arousal levels. On a cognitive level, records of self-talk (what persons say to themselves) were kept with emphasis on increasing the amount of positive self-talk, reducing negative self-talk, and using specific self-instructions (e.g., "stay calm" in tense situations). In addition, certain emotions such as anger or fear were identified, distinguished from one another, and used to probe how personal beliefs about certain events are related to behavior and emotions (e.g., subject was criticized by someone and then experienced anger).

Treatment methods were based in large part on theory and empirical work in behavioral self-management[34] and cognitive behavior modification.[35] Three related treatment strategies believed to be functional in all effective psychotherapeutic approaches[30] were used in designing techniques: (a) use of social modeling to demonstrate appropriate or desired behavior, (b) encouragement of persons to engage in new behavior, and (c) provision of prompt, corrective feedback about performance. Thus, group leaders used the group setting as a context to introduce new behavior, often modeling it themselves, followed by asking group members to practice it in the group, and then by offering corrective feedback to subjects as needed.

The treatment protocol began by teaching subjects how to identify a variety of overt TABP behaviors and characteristics (e.g., interrupting others, arguing tenaciously to win small points) first in others and then in themselves. Particular attention was initially paid to the experience of driving a car since the four major factors involved in the TABP (behavioral, physiologic, environmental, and cognitive) could readily be demonstrated in driving. Simultaneously, subjects learned to discriminate exaggerated physiologic, cognitive, and behavioral reactions to situations perceived as stressful as well as to develop physical and mental relaxation skills for use as alternative responses to stressful events. The initial primary focus on overt behavioral and environmental factors was gradually diminished over time so that cognitive factors, as the underpinnings of overt actions, began to receive more attention. Thus, common beliefs considered characteristic of the TABP were introduced, such as beliefs about oneself (e.g., distorted self-appraisal of personal qualities, overemphasis on contingent accomplishments as prime criterion for self-worth), beliefs about others (e.g., most people are basically hostile, extremely competitive, generally untrustworthy), and beliefs about life in general (e.g., career success depends on the TABP).

Treatment methods included lectures, slide presentations, and selected readings in order to provide an understanding of the theoretic rationale behind the concept of TABP and behavior change as well as to instruct and guide practice in the group settings. Liberal use was made of metaphors, aphorisms, diagrams, and audiotaped models of Type A and non-Type A behaviors and attitudes. Homework assignments were used between sessions to encourage further acquisition and generalization of understandings and skills derived from the group setting to everyday life.

Table 2 (page 109) is taken from a behavior practice manual called the *Drill Book* especially prepared for this study. Subjects were asked each month to focus on one behavior each day (e.g., in October, to practice eating more slowly on Thursdays) as well as to reflect daily on one quotation for each week (e.g., the fourth week in October reflect on "Habit is the hardiest of all the plants in human growth"). The need for the *Drill Book* became apparent during the first months of the study because initial compliance with homework assignments was found to be quite low.

TABLE 2: EXAMPLE FROM THE RECURRENT CORONARY PREVENTION PROJECT'S <u>DRILL BOOK</u> USED IN THE TYPE A BEHAVIORAL GROUP TREATMENT

<u>October</u>

Monday:	Set aside 30 minutes for yourself
Tuesday:	Practice smiling
Wednesday:	Practice removing your grimaces
Thursday:	Eat more slowly
Friday:	Recall memories for 10 minutes
Saturday:	Verbalize affection to spouse/children
Sunday:	Linger at table

1.* "The only future we can conceive is built upon the forward shadow of our past" - Proust.
2. "If you make the organization your life, you are defenseless against the inevitable disappointments" - Peter Drucker.
3. "The moment numeration ceases to be your servant, it becomes your tyrant" - Anonymous.
4. "Habit is the hardiest of all the plants in human growth" - Anonymous.

*Reflect on the first quote daily for the first week; the second daily for the second week, and so on.

Significantly, for the vast majority of subjects, the group became a special social environment in which new behaviors could be tried, peer and leader support and encouragement could be offered, and basic beliefs and perceptions of oneself and others could be seriously examined. Typically, the format for a 90-minute group session was as follows: (a) brief relaxation practice; (b) review and discussion of homework assignments, such as *Drill Book* readings or observations from the home or work environment; (c) introduction of new material, often the demonstration of a new skill (e.g., self-instructional sequence in anticipated stressful situations); (d) review of assignments for the next meeting; and (e) closing benediction. However, the group leader was always at liberty to rearrange the planned agenda contingent on problems and concerns that might be raised by group members. Often on such occasions, the group leader might employ group problem-solving to assist the person, coupled with using the group to provide emotional and social support.

RECENT TREATMENT OUTCOMES

Briefly, the main findings as of 1985 indicate that subjects in the combined cardiologic and Type A behavioral counseling treatment had a 3-year cumulative reinfarction rate of 7.2%, compared with 13.2% in subjects who received cardiologic counseling treatment only ($P < .005$), using the intention-to-treat principle (i.e., the entire initial cohort including dropouts). Subjects in the nontreatment comparison group had a 14.0% recurrence rate of infarction. Comparable figures for subjects who actively remained in treatment (i.e., did not drop out) after 3 years were 8.9%, 18.9%, and 17.1% ($P < .001$) for the cardiologic and Type A behavioral treatment, cardiologic treatment, and nontreatment comparison group, respectively. Hence, the total recurrence rate for subjects receiving the Type A behavioral counseling was almost 50% less than those receiving either cardiologic counseling or no special treatment.

In terms of reductions in TABP, patients remaining in the study during the first 3 years that received the behavioral counseling demonstrated significant reductions of TABP on both the participant questionnaire and the VSI. The mean change in the questionnaire scores at entry was from 2.7 ± 0.42 to 2.14 ± 0.39 at the end of the third year, a change of approximately 1-1/2 standard deviations ($P < .001$). The cardiologic counseling treatment also demonstrated a significant ($P < .05$) reduction - from 2.69 ± 0.42 to 2.40 ± 0.38. However, this reduction was significantly less than that observed in the Type A behavioral counseling treatment group ($P < .001$). Importantly, changes on the spouse and monitor questionnaires showed very comparable changes for those reported by subjects in the Type A behavioral counseling group, thus providing some outside corroboration of the self-reported changes.

The VSI scores for Type A treatment fell from 28.0 ± 11.9 at entry to 17.0 ± 8.3 during the third year ($P < .001$). In contrast, subjects in the cardiologic counseling treatment demonstrated a significant ($P < .05$) but more modest reduction (29.2 ± 12.2 to 23.1 ± 9.2). Again, reduction in the Type A treatment group was significantly greater than that observed in the cardiologic treatment group ($P < .001$).

What of the relationship between reduced TABP and reduced cardiac recurrences? To examine this question, 181 subjects were identified who had reduced their TABP score by at least one standard deviation on the participant questionnaire by the end of the first year. The cumulative second- and third-year cardiac recurrence rates of these 181 "high change" subjects was one-fourth (1.7% vs. 8.6%) that of persons who had failed to show significant reductions in TABP scores (i.e., changed less than one standard deviation) at the end of the first year ($P < .001$). Significant demographic or entry medical findings were not found (e.g., age, serum cholesterol level, past history of smoking, drug regimens, angina, complex arrhythmias, or congestive heart failure) between these groups that might account for differences in recurrence rates. Of the 181 persons showing marked TABP score reductions at the end of the first year and followed for the next 2 years, 90.6% ($N = 164$) were found to be enrolled in the combined Type A behavioral and cardiologic counseling treatment.

Differences were not found at 3 years between the Type A treatment versus the cardiologic treatment groups in terms of the number of subjects who had undergone bypass surgery (8.7% vs. 8.7%); the number taking various medications, such as beta blockers (29.9% vs. 26.6%), vasodilators (26.8% vs. 27.7%) and antiarrhythmics (12.2% vs. 11.5%); and the number suffering from congestive heart failure, hypertension, or arrhythmia. However, a significant reduction ($P < .05$) for the Type A behavioral counseling subjects was found in the symptoms of angina compared with cardiologic counseling only subjects (47.8% vs. 59.4%). Furthermore, subjects in both treatment groups had significantly ($P < .001$) reduced their serum cholesterol levels from entry values, from 264 ± 51.5 mg/dl to 237.6 ± 48.1 mg/dl for the Type A treatment group and from 259 ± 41.2 mg/dl to 235.4 ± 47.6 mg/dl for the cardiologic counseling group, a reduction of about one-half standard deviation from entry level, or 10%.

CONCLUSION

Results of the RCPP and of a few other intervention studies have been encouraging. For the first time, a controlled prospective study has demonstrated that alterations in TABP are associated with noteworthy (both statistically and clinically) reductions in recurrences of myocardial infarction. A basis for guarded optimism has been established, suggesting that other controlled studies focusing on the modification of TABP deserve careful consideration. Clearly, future studies should carefully consider how to assess the TABP, avoiding sole reliance on any self-report questionnaire and use of oversimplified category ratings (e.g., A_1, A_2, X, B). As conceptual and assessment studies progress in such areas as anger-hostility and physiologic hyper-reactivity, a further clarification of which features of TABP deserve treatment should emerge.[36] For now, it seems prudent to use comprehensive treatment protocols that focus on major TABP behaviors and characteristics. The continued use of small treatment groups seems highly warranted, especially since the groups are highly effective and efficient laboratories for learning and behavior change.

Careful consideration, however, is needed in the selection and training of therapeutic group leaders. The typical composition of post-infarction groups, compared with those individual patients commonly seen in private psychiatric/psychologic practice, often required leaders to cope with patients that are highly challenging, often very hostile, and at times, extremely skeptical. Group leaders must not only provide a well-structured and planned session, but understand that their own Type A behavior, if not recognized and clearly acknowledged, can undermine the entire treatment program.[29] An effective group leader succeeds as much by personal example as by any particular method. Finally, the need to acknowledge good health and well-being as an ongoing integration of physiologic, behavioral, cognitive, and environmental factors appears to be useful. Too often, the patient as a person feels ignored, if not diminished, when treatment focuses exclusively on physiologic factors, and casual advice is at times offered about the need to "take it easy."

REFERENCES

1. Osler W: *Lectures on Angina Pectoris and Allied States*. New York, Appleton, 1897.
2. Weiner H: *Psychobiology and Human Disease*. New York, Elsevier-North Holland, 1977.

3. Friedman M: *Pathogenesis of Coronary Artery Disease.* New York, McGraw-Hill, 1969.
4. Friedman M, Thoresen CE, Gill JJ: Type A behavior: Its role, detection and alteration in patients with Ischemic heart disease, in Hurst JW (ed): *Update V - The Heart.* New York, McGraw-Hill, 1981:81-100.
5. Dunbar HF: *Psychosomatic Diagnosis.* New York, Hoeber, 1943.
6. Menninger KA, Menninger WC: Psychoanalytic observations in cardiac disorders. *Am Heart J* 1936;11:10.
7. Price VA: *Type A Behavior: A Model for Research and Practice.* New York, Academic Press, 1982.
8. Thoresen CE, Ohman A: The type A behavior pattern: A person-environment interaction perspective, in Magnusson D, Ohman A (eds): *Psychopathology: An Interaction Perspective.* New York, Academic Press, 1985.
9. Suinn RM: Intervention with type A behavior. *J Consult Clin Psychol* 1982;50:933-949.
10. Carruthers ME: Aggression and atheroma. *Lancet* 1969;2:1170.
11. Friedman M, Byers SO, Rosenman RH: Effect of unsaturated fats upon lipemia and conjunctival circulation. *JAMA* 1965;193:882.
12. Friedman M, Rosenman RH, Byers SO: Serum lipids and conjunctival circulation after fat ingestion in men exhibiting type A behavior pattern. *Circulation* 1964;29:874.
13. Caffrey B: Behavior patterns and personality characteristics related to prevalence rates of coronary heart disease in American monks. *J Chronic Dis* 1969;22:93.
14. Blumenthal JA, Williams RB Jr, Kong Y, Schanberg SM, Thompson LW: Type A behavior pattern and coronary atherosclerosis. *Circulation* 1978;58:534-559.
15. Friedman M, Manwaring JH, Rosenman RH, Donlon G, Ortega D, Grube SM: Instantaneous and sudden death: Clinical and pathological differentiation in coronary artery disease. *JAMA* 1973;225:1319-1322.
16. Glass DC: *Behavior Pattern, Stress and Coronary Disease.* Hillsdale, NJ, Erlbaum, 1977.
17. Haynes SG, Feinleib M, Kannel WB: The relationship of psychosocial factors to coronary heart disease in the Framingham Study. III. Eight-year incidence of coronary heart disease. *Am J Epidemiol* 1980;111:37-58.
18. Rosenman RH, Brand RJ, Jenkins CD, Friedman M, Straus R, Wurm M: Coronary heart disease in the Western

Collaborative Group Study: Final follow-up experience of 8 1/2 years. *JAMA* 1975;23:872-877.
19. Review Panel of Coronary-Prone Behavior and Coronary Heart Disease: A critical review. *Circulation* 1981; 63:1199-1215.
20. Matthews KA: Psychological perspectives on the Type A behavior pattern. *Psychol Bull* 1982;91:293-323.
21. Thoresen CE, Telch MJ, Eagleston JR: Approaches to altering the type A behavior pattern. *Psychosomatics* 1981;22:472-482.
22. Matthews KA, Krantz DS, Dembroski TM, MacDougall JM: The unique and common variance in the Structured Interview and the Jenkins Activity Survey measures of the Type A behavior pattern. *J Pers Soc Psych* 1982;42:303-313.
23. Levenkron JD, Cohen J, Mueller H, Fisher E: Modifying the Type A coronary-prone behavior pattern. *J Consult Clin Psychol* 1983;51:192-204.
24. Suinn RM: The cardiac stress management program for Type A patients. *Cardiac Rehabilitation* 1975;5:13-15.
25. Suinn RM, Bloom LJ: Anxiety management training for Pattern A behavior. *J Behav Med* 1978;1:25-35.
26. Jenni MA, Wollersheim JP: Cognitive therapy, stress management training, and the Type A behavior pattern. *Cogn Ther Res* 1979;3:61-73.
27. Roskies E, Spevack M, Surkis A, Cohen G, Gilman S: Changing the coronary-prone (Type A) behavior pattern in a nonclinical population. *J Behav Med* 1978;1:201-216.
28. Friedman M, Thoresen CE, Gill JJ, Ulmer D, Powell L, Thompson L, Price VA, Elek SR, Rabin DD, Piaget G, Dixon TR, Bourg E, Levy RA, Tasto DL: Feasibility of altering Type A behavior pattern in post-myocardial infarction patients. *Circulation* 1982;66:83-92.
29. Thoresen CE, Friedman M, Gill JJ, Ulmer DK: The Recurrent Coronary Prevention Project: Some preliminary findings. *Acta Med Scand* 1982;660(Suppl):172-192.
30. Friedman M, Thoresen CE, Gill JJ, Powell LH, Ulmer D, Thompson L, Price VA, Rabin DD, Breall WS, Dixon T, Levy R, Bourg E: Alteration of type A behavior and reduction in cardiac recurrences in post-myocardial infarction subjects. *Am Heart J* 1984;108:237-248.
31. Powell LH, Friedman M, Thoresen CE, Gill JJ, Ulmer D: Can the type A behavior pattern be altered after myocardial infarction? A second year report from the Recurrent Coronary Prevention Project. *Psychosom Med* 1984;46:293-313.

32. Chesney MA, Eagleston JR, Rosenman RH: The type A Structured Interview: A behavioral assessment in the rough. *Journal of Behavioral Assessment* 1980;2:255-272.
33. Thoresen CE: Overview: Strategies for health enhancement, in Matarazzo JD, Weiss S, Herd JA, Miller N, Weiss S (eds): *Behavioral Health: A Handbook of Health Enhancement and Disease Prevention.* New York, Wiley, 1984;297-307.
34. Thoresen CE, Mahoney MJ; *Behavioral Self-Control.* New York, Holt, Rinehart and Winston, 1974.
35. Meichenbaum D: *Cognitive Behavior Modification.* New York, Plenum, 1977.
36. Chesney MA, Rosenman RH (eds): *Anger and Hostility in Cardiovascular and Behavioral Disorders.* New York, Hemisphere/McGraw-Hill, 1985.

8

Behavioral Effects of Beta Blockers: Reduction of Anxiety, Acute Stress, and Type A Behavior*

Lynn A. Durel, David S. Krantz, John F. Eisold, and Jeffrey D. Lazar

INTRODUCTION

Since the introduction of the beta-adrenoreceptor antagonists and their wide use for cardiovascular disorders, a variety of both desirable and unwanted psychologic effects of these drugs have been observed.[1,2] One of the most commonly noted beneficial effects has been the reduction of reported anxiety among certain patient groups. These drugs have also been studied as anxiolytic agents for healthy subjects under acutely stressful circumstances (e.g., performing before an audience, dental surgery) accompanied by severe somatic manifestations of arousal.[3,4] In addition, recent reports[5,6] suggest that chronic beta-blocker therapy may also have effects in decreasing the intensity of Type A (coronary-prone) behavior.

Most pharmacologic attempts to reduce stress-related cardiovascular changes have concentrated on processes at the level of the central nervous system (CNS). Although actions of beta blockers in the CNS have been amply substantiated,[1] many of the psychologic effects are thought

---

*Preparation of this chapter was assisted by NIH grant HL31514 and USUHS grants R07233 and C07562. Opinions expressed reflect those of the authors and do not represent those of the USUHS, Naval Hospital, Bethesda, or the Department of Defense.

to result from blockade of receptors at the reacting end organs. Specifically, clinically relevant anxiolytic effects may be produced by suppressing somatic symptoms of anxiety or stress and their feedback to the CNS. This chapter will focus on current research concerning the psychologic and behavioral effects of beta blockers; however, in order to understand how these agents affect concomitants of anxiety, stress, and emotional behavior, we begin with a brief review of their pharmacology and physiologic effects.

PHARMACOLOGIC PROPERTIES AND PHYSIOLOGIC EFFECTS

Beta blockers are structurally similar to the body's adrenergic neurotransmitters, norepinephrine and epinephrine, but especially to those sympathomimetic agonists that preferentially activate the beta receptors. As they competitively inhibit binding at the beta subset of adrenergic receptors, they typically display their greatest physiologic effects during periods of intense sympathetic nervous system (SNS) activity (i.e., when the transmitters with which they compete for receptor sites would otherwise exert their maximal effects). In other words, their effects are relatively slight when sympathetic activity is minimal (during rest) and greater when the SNS responds to physical or psychologic demands.[7]

The most clinically relevant actions of beta blockers are on the cardiovascular system; hence, their primary use is for the treatment of hypertension, angina pectoris, and cardiac arrhythmias and for the prevention of reinfarction.[8,9] Although the focus of study of these drugs has been on their cardiovascular effects, the development of newer agents has resulted in an appreciation of the complexity of action of this group of drugs.[8,10,11] For example, the efficacy of beta blockers with intrinsic sympathomimetic activity (ISA) strengthens the conclusion that their antihypertensive actions cannot be attributed primarily to beta blockade of the heart.[7,12]

In addition to cardiovascular activity, numerous other physiologic functions are beta-adrenergically mediated. For example, lipolysis is increased by stimulation of beta-1 receptors. Beta-2 receptors, located in smooth muscle and glands, mediate bronchiolar dilation, glycogenolysis, gluconeogenesis, renin secretion, and skeletal muscle vasodilation. Responses to adrenergic impulses are not limited to the effector organs mentioned here, and other effects of beta blockade also occur that are beyond the scope of this chapter.[7]

PROPERTIES OF BETA BLOCKERS

Since two types of beta adrenoceptors have been identified,[13] it has become common practice to categorize these agents according to their preferential sites of action. Those that block cardiostimulation and lipolysis are categorized as beta-1, those that block vasodilation, beta-2.

It is important to point out that beta selectivity is a relative phenomenon. That is, at low doses of a drug, one type of antagonism (usually beta-1) may predominate, whereas at higher doses, this differential action is lost and both receptor types are blocked.[8,10]

Not all effects of this class of drugs are caused by beta blockade per se. Other properties that may influence drug effects include membrane stabilizing activity (MSA) and ISA (or partial agonist activity). Membrane stabilizing activity results in local-anesthetic or quinidine-like effects on cell membranes; this activity is unrelated to beta blockade, occurs only in high drug doses, and is not believed to be clinically relevant.[8] Intrinsic sympathomimetic activity is a less understood property of several beta blockers that provide partial agonist activity while also inhibiting binding of agonists and transmitters. These drugs cause less decrease in resting heart rate than antagonists without ISA, but block equally at high levels of SNS activity.[8]

Finally, the issue of lipophilicity has been raised in discussion of the sites of action of beta blockers. Drugs that are lipid soluble are better able to penetrate the blood-brain barrier, thereby accumulating in brain tissue to a greater degree than do those that are more water soluble. This ability of the lipid-soluble beta blockers might be related to side effects that are thought to be centrally mediated, for example, nightmares and depression.[8,11,14] Table 1 (page 120) shows the relative cardioselectivity, lipophilicity, MSA, and ISA of Federal Drug Administration-approved or soon-to-be-approved beta blockers.

TABLE 1: COMPARATIVE PHARMACOLOGY OF BETA BLOCKERS

Drug	Cardio-selective?	Equivalent Doses*	H/L	ISA	MSA
Propranolol	No	-	L	-	++
Atenolol	Yes	50 mg qd	H	-	-
Metoprolol	Yes	50 mg bid	L	-	+/-
Nadolol	No	80 mg qd	H	-	-
Oxprenolol	No	40 mg bid	L	+/++	+
Pindolol	No	10 mg tid**	L	+++	+/-
Timolol	No	10 mg bid	L	+/-	-

*Equivalent to propranolol 40 mg bid.
**Average value obtained from several sources.

H = hydrophilic; L = lipophilic; ISA = intrinsic sympathomimetic activity; MSA = membrane stabilizing activity.

(Adapted from Frishman WH.[48])

PSYCHOLOGIC EFFECTS

ANXIETY REDUCTION

First reported by Granville-Grossman and Turner[15] with propranolol, the anxiolytic effect of beta blockers in chronically anxious patients has been repeatedly observed. However, when compared with other anxiolytic drugs such as the minor tranquilizers (e.g., diazepam), beta antagonists are probably most effective primarily in patients whose anxiety is characterized by bodily complaints.[16,17] In other words, when patients describe their anxiety more in terms of palpitations and tremor than as worry and mental tension, their anxiety is likely to be reduced with a beta blocker. When psychic symptoms predominate, beta blockers are considered much less effective than benzodiazepines.[1,3] There is some evidence, however, that psychic symptoms may be responsive to prolonged therapy with high-dose propranolol.[18]

Although there is a general anxiolytic effect for even the newer beta blockers, the complexity of their pharmacologic actions and physiologic and psychologic effects contributes to confusion about mechanisms responsible for these effects.

EFFECTS DURING SITUATIONAL STRESS

Considerable evidence has shown not only that beta blockers can alleviate some chronic anxiety conditions, but also that they are useful in decreasing anxiety in certain acute stress situations. These effects have been demonstrated in healthy people, in patients with cardiovascular disease, and under conditions of both acute and chronic drug administration.[1-4]

In healthy subjects, beta blockers blunt the increases in cardiovascular activity and anxiety that accompany certain stressful activities such as public speaking, examinations, race car driving, musical performance, and oral surgery.[1,2,17-20] In cardiac patients and in hypertensive patients, chronic beta blockade reduces the occurrence of certain emotional and speech characteristics and attenuates the cardiovascular responses of patients undergoing a challenging interview.[5,6,21] Recently, the anxiolytic effect of beta blockade in a public speaking situation has also been reported for post-myocardial infarction patients.[22] Few studies have compared different beta blockers in acute anxiety-arousing situations. However, anxiolytic effects have been reported for a variety of beta blockers regardless of whether they are lipophilic and able to penetrate the blood-brain barrier.

Less consistent are the effects of beta blockers on human performance during stress and nonstressful circumstances.[1] Some reviewers conclude that beta blockers exert their anxiolytic effect without significant impairment in cognitive or psychologic performance,[11,23] whereas others report poorer performance or increased variability with some beta blockers on tests of reaction time[23-25] and memory.[26] Still others have concluded that the occasionally observed decrement in several psychomotor functions is indicative not of a depressant effect on CNS function but of an action of skeletal muscle.[2] In this regard, when situational stress leads to a decrement in performance, which in turn, increases anxiety further (e.g., the anxiety-induced tremor experienced by some string musicians during public performance), reduction of anxiety or tremor by beta blockade apparently leads to improved performance.[1,18,20]

It should be noted that a shortcoming of many of the studies designed to evaluate the presumed central effects of drugs on performance has been the failure to rule out the possibility that the occurrence of decrements was due to peripheral effects. Another shortcoming has been the lack of control groups adequate to establish that the tasks used are sensitive to CNS effects. Therefore, many beta-blocker studies of performance may not have been adequate tests of their degree of central action.[11] In addition, since the majority of studies of performance effects of beta blockers have involved acute drug administration, the effects of chronic beta blockade on performance and other behavioral and attitudinal parameters have not been clearly elucidated. For example, one study reported a decrement in complex reaction time only when propranolol was given acutely; after 4 weeks, there was no difference in complex reaction time between subjects receiving propranolol and those receiving placebo.[24] On the other hand, some performance decrements have even been reported with chronic administration of the hydrophilic agent atenolol.[25]

Although definite conclusions cannot be drawn at this time regarding the types and levels of performance effects attributable to various beta blockers, the available data suggest that these drugs generally do result in anxiety reduction, but have variable effects on performance in stressful situations. In addition, recent evidence[27] suggests that there may be performance deficits resulting from disease states such as hypertension that might be improved by pharmacologic treatment (e.g., with beta blockers).

MECHANISMS INVOLVED IN ANXIETY REDUCTION WITH BETA BLOCKADE

The precise mechanisms by which the anxiolytic and stress-reducing effects of beta blockade occur are not entirely clear. A central site of action is often assumed, especially when effects on mood or behavior are associated with a lipophilic beta blocker.[28] Although all the commonly used beta blockers penetrate the CNS to some extent, they vary widely in degree of penetration. It appears that this can be explained largely on the basis of lipid solubility, although other factors (amount of free drug in plasma and degree of ionization) may also play minor roles.[1,2] Protein binding influences the extent to which drugs are free to leave the plasma and enter the cerebrospinal fluid (CSF);[1] consequently, the CSF concentrations of these drugs differ from their brain tissue concentrations.[14] Since beta receptors are thought to be on cell surfaces, CSF concentrations as well as brain concentrations may influence any beta-blocker activity in the brain.[29] These drugs may also act at other receptor sites, for example, that for serotonin (5HT), possibly resulting in a centrally mediated antianxiety effect.[30] Finally, the membrane stabilizing action exhibited by some beta blockers administered at very high doses could be responsible for a nonspecific depressant effect in the CNS.[11]

It is important to note that penetration of beta-blocking drugs into the CNS is not sufficient to prove that the drugs have a central action. In fact, most reviewers[2,7,17] believe that the peripheral action of beta blockers is sufficient to account for their anxiety-reducing effects. This mechanism may involve the role of information processing concerning peripheral sympathetic responses on the subjective experience of emotion.

Peripheralist views of emotion (e.g., James-Lange, Schachter-Singer) suggest that the subjective experience of anxiety is a result of a sequence of physiologic events beginning with sympathetic stimulation leading to arousal manifestations, such as palpitation and tremor. The perception, cognitive interpretation, or automatic processing of these responses acts to reinforce the psychic elements of anxiety. Based on this interpretation, beta blockade inhibits peripheral physiologic responses, interrupts the somatic-psychic interaction, and thus reduces anxiety.[2-4,16,21]

This peripheral feedback explanation for the anxiolytic effects of beta blockers receives support from several sources. First, there is evidence that beta blockers such as atenolol (which does not readily penetrate the brain) may be as effective in reducing anxiety as propranolol.[2,7] Thus, when given in acute doses, beta blockers with little access to either the brain or the CSF have anxiolytic effects.[2,4,20] Second, beta blockers are most effective in patients who exhibit anxiety characterized particularly by somatic symptoms, such as palpitations and tremor, rather than in those who characterize their distress or anxiety in terms of purely cognitive or psychic terms, such as worrisome or fearful thoughts.[16] However, the relative contributions of peripheral and central mechanisms to the anxiolytic and other psychologic effects of beta blockers continue to be controversial.[1,2,4,11,14]

ANXIOLYTIC EFFECTS OF BETA BLOCKERS VERSUS BENZODIAZEPINES IN CARDIAC PATIENTS

Anxiety reduction by beta blockade in cardiac patients can be contrasted with the anxiolytic effect of the benzodiazepines. Administered orally, the traditional anxiolytic drugs do not have any direct cardiovascular effects.[31] However, they may have some beneficial effects on hemodynamic activity in anxious cardiac patients.[31-33] Diazepam and other benzodiazepines are thought to interrupt the anxiety-cardiac responsivity loop by central tranquilization, that is, by inhibiting the activation of the sympathetic-adrenomedullary axis during the anxiety process.[31] This dampening of activity in the efferent arm may prevent the cardiovascular hyperresponsiveness associated with anxiety. It has been suggested that anxiety reduction with benzodiazepines in cardiac patients may be associated with a lowering of myocardial oxygen consumption and a reduction in the incidence of angina pectoris and myocardial infarction.[32,33] This central anxiolytic mechanism proposed for the minor tranquilizers, then, contrasts with the proposed peripheral mechanism for beta blockers. With the traditional anxiolytics, reduction of anxiety has a beneficial effect on cardiovascular function; with the beta blockers, reduction in cardiovascular function leads to decreases in anxiety. Although these processes may be logically and empirically separable, both probably contribute to physiologic and psychologic relaxation.

TYPE A BEHAVIOR: ASSESSMENT AND PHYSIOLOGIC CORRELATES

The Type A behavior pattern, implicated as an independent risk factor for ischemic heart disease (IHD), is characterized by excessive competitive drive, impatience, hostility, and energetic speech mannerisms.[34,35] Assessment of Type A behavior using a structured interview heavily weights speech stylistics and the subject's manner of responding. Type A behavior can be measured in a face-to-face interview[36] or with the questionnaire developed by Jenkins.[34,37] The structured interview seems to be a better predictor of IHD than the questionnaire and also has a stronger correlation with psychophysiologic responses to stress.[38,39] This type of interview can be reliably scored for speech stylistics (loud/explosive, rapid,

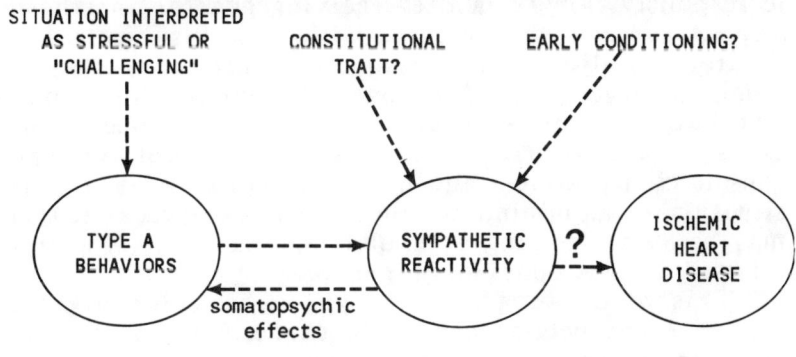

Figure 1. Model illustrating possible relationships between Type A behavior and sympathetic nervous system reactivity. (Adapted from Krantz & Durel[21])

potential-for-hostility, etc.) as well as for categories of Type A and content or self-descriptive responses of the individual.

Type A behaviors are thought to be accompanied by potentially pathogenic sympathetic neuroendocrine and hemodynamic responses. Many studies have demonstrated larger increases in blood pressure, heart rate, or plasma catecholamine levels in Type A than in Type B individuals in challenging situations.[38-39] Therefore, attempts to explain the link between Type A individuals and IHD suggest that situations perceived as stressful or challenging elicit Type A behavior in susceptible individuals and, in turn, evoke physiologic responses (i.e., sympathetic and sympathoadrenal discharge) that act on the cardiovascular system to promote or precipitate IHD (Figure 1). However, in addition to the effects of situationally elicited psychologic factors on sympathetic nervous system responsivity, there is some tentative evidence that sympathetic responsiveness might also influence manifestations of Type A behavior.[5,6,21] This evidence has suggested that elements of the Type A behavior pattern may be decreased by beta blockers.

POSSIBLE EFFECTS OF BETA BLOCKERS ON TYPE A BEHAVIOR

Results of two studies of coronary artery bypass graft surgery suggest that Type A behavior exhibited by cardiac patients may in part reflect an underlying sympathetic responsivity.[40,41] While receiving general anesthesia, Type A subjects, as compared with Type B subjects, have greater systolic blood pressure increases over hospital admission levels, a finding that was related to intraoperative but not to pre-operative increases.[41] Since the increased cardiovascular responses were observed when conscious mediation - and hence perception of a stressful situation - was minimized, these results suggest that there may be an underlying psychobiologic basis for interview-assessed Type A behavior (Figure 1).

This would suggest that Type A behavior might be suppressed by beta-adrenergic blockade, with its attendant decrease in sympathetic responsiveness. Two preliminary studies provide support for the effects of chronic beta blockade on Type A behavior. In one study,[5] a correlational analysis compared behavioral and psychophysiologic characteristics of coronary patients receiving propranolol as part of their medical program with those of patients not receiving the beta blockers. Results indicated that propranolol-treated patients displayed less Type A speech and behavioral stylistics than did patients not taking propranolol. Such effects were not found among patients receiving diuretics, nitrates, or central nervous system active drugs (e.g., benzodiazepines). The aspects of Type A behavior that were reduced in patients receiving beta blockers included loud/explosive, rapid/accelerated speech and potential for hostility, not the patients' descriptions of themselves as competitive, impatient, and so on. Since these data are correlational, it cannot be concluded that propranolol specifically caused a lessening of Type A behavior. However, the data are suggestive, since the effects were still present after controlling for a variety of possibly confounding factors, such as age, presence of symptoms, and severity of disease.

A second study that provided evidence that chronic beta-blocker therapy might decrease Type A behavior resulted from a recent experiment in which one group of hypertensive patients received atenolol and the other received a thiazide diuretic.[6] After receiving medication for over 4 weeks, the beta-blocker group, but not the controls, showed a decrease in intensity of Type A behavior as assessed by structured interview. By attenuation of sympathetic reactivity with atenolol, behavioral manifestations of Type A behavior appeared to be lessened. However, this study was not placebo controlled, and the diuretic was associated with some increases in Type A behavior characteristics. Hence, placebo-controlled investigations of the Type A-reducing phenomenon are necessary to confirm the suggested effects of beta blockers on such behavior. Moreover, since the precise pathophysiologic mechanisms responsible for the associations of Type A behavior with IHD are not yet known, further research is needed before recommending beta blockers for the management of coronary risk conferred by Type A behavior.

UNDESIRABLE PSYCHOLOGIC AND BEHAVIORAL EFFECTS OF BETA BLOCKERS

In addition to the psychologic effects previously described - many of which may be considered beneficial - it must be emphasized that unwanted psychologic and behavioral effects of beta blockers have been observed. Side effects such as fatigue, depression, nightmares, and disturbances of sleep and sexual function have been reported.[1,3,7,42,43] Although it has been suggested that these side effects may be less with the hydrophilic and cardioselective beta blockers,[28,43] it remains unclear whether the side effects are actually attributable to beta blockade per se or to other specific properties of the drugs.[7] Although large-scale studies such as the Beta Blocker Heart Attack Trial[9] have reported minimal frequency of occurrence of these adverse effects, the clinician treating hypertensive or post-myocardial infarction patients has no doubt noted that those effects occur with sufficient frequency to cause considerable discomfort and often noncompliance with drug therapy.

In light of recent speculation that stress-related catecholamine release may play a role in the pathophysiology of IHD,[32,38,39] we note that some studies have reported greater increases in plasma catecholamines during exercise and mental stress in subjects receiving certain beta blockers.[19,44-46] However, other studies have obtained opposite results,[45,47] and further research is needed concerning the effects of acute and chronic beta blockade on plasma catecholamines.

CONCLUSIONS AND IMPLICATIONS

We have described some of the actions and effects of beta blockers, with particular emphasis on evidence that they decrease anxiety, situational stress, and Type A behavior. However, anxiolytic effects seem most pronounced in patients who are disturbed by somatic manifestations of anxiety or stress.

Certain emotion-related psychologic and behavioral changes occurring in cardiac patients receiving beta blockers are thought to reflect the inhibition of beta-adrenergic responses to sympathetic nervous system activity. For those cardiac patients who display high levels of SNS activity and who are disturbed by somatic symptoms, beta blockers may provide a means for controlling pathophysiologic mechanisms and perhaps the psychobiologic effects of stress, with relatively few detrimental effects on performance. Thus, beta blockers have been recommended for chronic therapy for patients with hypertension, arrhythmias, a history of myocardial infarction, angina pectoris, or a host of other disorders.[1,4,7,48] The variety of actions exhibited by the drugs in this class makes it difficult to generalize about their effects but allows for considerable individualization of drug treatment. For example, cardiac patients experiencing intolerable side effects with propranolol therapy may well tolerate atenolol. Conversely, if anxiety persists during treatment with a less central nervous system-active beta blocker, it may be relieved by one with a wider range of pharmacologic actions.

SUMMARY

Beta-adrenergic blocking drugs have a variety of psychologic and behavioral effects. Among those effects considered beneficial, decreases in anxiety and Type A behavior and improved psychologic reactions to acutely stressful situations have been observed. The somatic manifestations of these conditions appear to be reduced more effectively by beta blockade than are cognitive or attitudinal manifestations. Because of this, the emotion-related influences of these drugs are primarily thought to reflect the inhibition of peripheral beta-adrenergic responses. This chapter reviews evidence for these effects and describes cautions regarding unwanted psychologic and behavioral side effects of beta blockers with different pharmacologic properties. For cardiac patients disturbed by somatic symptoms, beta blockers may provide a means for reducing psychobiologic effects of stress, with relatively little impact on task performance.

REFERENCES

1. Patel L, Turner P: Central actions of beta-adrenoceptor blocking drugs in man. *Med Res Rev* 1981;1:387-410.
2. Middlemiss DN, Buxton DA, Greenwood DT: Beta-adrenoceptor antagonists in psychiatry and neurology. *Pharmacol Ther* 1981;12:419-437.
3. Frishman WH, Razin A, Swencionis C, et al: Beta-adrenoceptor blockade in anxiety states: New approach to therapy? *Cardiovas Rev Rep* 1981;2:447-459.
4. Noyes R: Beta-blocking drugs and anxiety. *Psychosomatics* 1982;23:155-170.
5. Krantz D, Durel LA, Davia JE, et al: Propranolol medication among coronary patients: Relationship to type A behavior and cardiovascular response. *J Human Stress* 1982;8(3)4-12.
6. Schmieder R, Friedrich G, Neus H, et al: The influence of beta-blockers on cardiovascular reactivity and type A behavior pattern in hypertensives. *Psychosom Med* 1983;45:417-423.
7. Weiner N: Drugs that inhibit adrenergic nerves and block adrenergic receptors, in Goodman-Gilman AG, Goodman LS, Gilman A (eds): *Goodman and Gilman's The Pharmacological Basis of Therapeutics*, Ed 6. New York, Macmillan, 1980:176-210.
8. Frishman WH: ß-adrenoceptor antagonists: New drugs and new indications. *N Engl J Med* 1981;9:500-506.
9. ß-Blocker Heart Attack Study Group: The ß-blocker heart attack trial. *JAMA* 1981;246:2073-2074.
10. Andersson KE; Adrenoceptors: Classification, activation, and blockade by drugs. *Postgrad Med J* 1980;56(suppl 2):7-16.
11. Turner P: Beta-adrenoceptor blocking drugs and the central nervous system in man, in Turner P, Shand D (eds): *Recent Advances in Clinical Pharmacology*. London, Churchill & Livingston, 1983:223-234.
12. Scriven AJ, Lewis PJ: Beta-adrenergic blocking drugs in the treatment of hypertension. *Pharmacol Ther* 1983;20:95-131.
13. Lands AM, Luduena FP, Buzzo HJ: Differentiation of receptor systems responsive to isoproterenol. *Life Sci* 1967;6:2241.

14. Neil-Dwyer G, Bartlett J, McAinsh J, et al: ß-adrenoceptor blockers and the blood-brain barrier. *Br J Clin Pharmacol* 1981;12:549-553.
15. Granville-Grossman K, Turner P: The effect of propranolol on anxiety. *Lancet* 1966;1:788.
16. Tyrer PJ, Lader MH: Response to propranolol and diazepam in somatic and psychic anxiety. *Br Med J* 1974;14-16.
17. Tyrer PJ: *The Role of Bodily Feelings in Anxiety.* London, Oxford University Press, 1976.
18. Suzman MM: Use of Beta-adrenergic receptor blocking agents in psychiatry, in Palmer GC (ed): *Neuropharmacology of Central Nervous System and Behavioral Disorders.* New York, Academic Press, 1981;340-391.
19. Brisse B, Tetsch P, Jacobs W, et al: ß-adrenoceptor blockade in stress due to oral surgery. *Br J Clin Pharmacol* 1982;13:4218-4278.
20. Neftel KA, Adler RH, Kapelli L, et al: Stage fright in musicians: A model illustrating the effect of beta-blockers. *Psychosom Med* 1982;44:461-469.
21. Krantz DS, Durel LA: Psychobiological substrates of the type A behavior pattern. *Health Psychology* 1983;2:393-411.
22. Gatchel RJ, Gafney FA, Smith J: Reduction of stress in post-MI patients (abstract). *Psychophysiology* 1983; 20:442.
23. Landauer AA, Pocock DA, Prott FW: Effects of atenolol and propranolol on human performance and subjective feelings. *Psychopharmacology* 1979;60:211-215.
24. Broadhurst AD: The effect of propranolol on human performance. *Aviat Space Environ Med* 1980;51:176-179.
25. Salem SA, McDevitt DG: Central effects of beta-adrenoceptor antagonists. *Clin Pharmacol Ther* 1983;33:52-57.
26. Solomon S, Hotchkiss E, Saravay SM, et al: Impairment of memory function by antihypertensive medication. *Arch Gen Psychiatry* 1982;40:1109-1112.
27. Miller RE, Shapiro AP, King HE, et al: Effect of antihypertensive treatment on the behavioral consequences of elevated blood pressure. *Hypertension* 1984;6:202-208.
28. Cruickshank JM: The clinical importance of cardioselectivity and lipophilicity in beta blockers. *Am Heart J* 1980;100:160-178.
29. Brunner H: Observations of the pharmacology of the beta-blockers, in Kielholz P (ed): *Beta-Blockers and the*

Central Nervous System. Baltimore, University Park Press, 1976:11-20.
30. Middlemiss DN, Blakeborough L, Leather SP: Direct evidence for an interaction of beta-adrenergic blockers with the 5-HT receptor. *Nature* 1977;267:289-290.
31. Sigg EB: The pharmacological approaches to cardiac stress, in Eliot RS (ed): *Stress and the Heart.* New York, Futura, 1974.
32. Eliot RS: *Stress and the Major Cardiovascular Disorders.* New York, Futura, 1979.
33. Wheatley D (ed): *Stress and the Heart.* New York, Raven Press, 1977.
34. Blumenthal JA: Psychological assessment in cardiac rehabilitation. *J Cardiac Rehabil* 1985;5:208-215.
35. Thoresen CE, Friedman M, Powell LH, et al: Altering the type A behavior pattern in post-infarction patients. *J Cardiac Rehabil* 1985;5:258-266.
36. Rosenman RH: The interview method of assessment of the coronary-prone behavior pattern, in Dembroski TM, Weiss SM, Shields JL, et al (eds): *Coronary-Prone Behavior.* New York, Springer-Verlag, 1978.
37. Jenkins CD, Zyzanski SJ, Rosenman RH: Progress toward validation of a computer scored test for the type A coronary prone behavior pattern. *Psychosom Med* 1971;33:192-202.
38. Matthews KA: Psychological perspectives on the type A behavior pattern. *Psychol Bull* 1982;91:293-323.
39. Dembroski TM, MacDougall JM, Shields JL, et al: Components of the Type A coronary-prone behavior pattern and cardiovascular response to psychomotor performance challenge. *J Behav Med* 1978;11:159-176.
40. Kahn JP, Kornfeld DS, Frank KA, et al: Type A behavior and blood pressure during coronary artery bypass surgery. *Psychosom Med* 1980;42:407-414.
41. Krantz DS, Arabian JM, Davia JE, et al: Type A behavior and coronary artery bypass surgery: Intraoperative blood pressure and perioperative complications. *Psychosom Med* 1982;44:273-284.
42. Moss HB, Procci WR: Sexual dysfunction associated with oral hypertensive medications: A critical survey of the literature. *Gen Hosp Psychiatry* 1982;4:121-129.
43. Lazar J, Eisold J, Gadson I, et al: Recognition and management of antihypertensive drug side effects (abstract). *Clin Pharmacol Ther* 1984;35:254.
44. Dimsdale JE, Hartley LH, Ruskin J, Greenblatt DJ, LaBrie R: The effect of beta blockade on plasma cate-

cholamine levels after psychological and exercise stress. *Am J Cardiol* 1984;54:182-185.

45. Trap-Jensen J, Carlsen JE, Hartling OJ, et al: ß-adrenoceptor blockade and psychic stress in man: A comparison of the acute effects of labetol, metoprolol, pindolol, and propranolol on plasma levels of adrenaline and noradrenaline. *Br J Clin Pharmacol* 1982;13:3918-3958.

46. Bonelli J: Stress, catecholamines and beta-blockade. *Acta Med Scand* 1982;660:214-218.

47. Taggart P, Carruthers M, Summerville W: Electrocardiogram, plasma catecholamines and lipids, and their modification by oxprenolol when speaking before an audience. *Lancet* 1973;2:341-346.

48. Frishman WH: *Clinical Pharmacology of the Beta-Adrenoreceptor Blocking Drugs.* New York, Appleton Century-Crofts, 1980.

9

Psychologic and Social Outcomes Following Coronary Artery Bypass Surgery*

Julaine Kinchla and Theodore Weiss

This chapter reviews work published since 1980 concerning the psychologic and social outcomes following coronary artery bypass graft surgery (CABGS). First, employment patterns before and after surgery will be reviewed, then some variables that help predict these patterns will be considered. Next, we will describe other social and psychologic outcomes and conclude with a general discussion.

EMPLOYMENT STATUS: OUTCOME STATISTICS

A major psychosocial variable in the evaluation of CABGS is whether or not the patient returns to work. The importance of this variable is underscored by the large number of studies that have focused on employment status. One investigator explains:

> Return to work after major cardiac surgery is an important indicator of functional benefit to the patient and social benefit to the community for the resources expended. Most adults define their personal worth to some degree by their ability to fulfill a socially useful occupational role and find much of their interpersonal support and satisfaction at the workplace.[1]

---

*Supported in part by NIH Grant HL31514. Also, the authors gratefully acknowledge the help of Linda Levy in preparing the manuscript.

Bypass Surgery: Psychologic and Social Outcomes

Excellent reviews of work status following CABGS conducted before 1980 are presented by Oberman and associates[2] and Doehrman.[3] A review that provides a more comprehensive international perspective is the analysis and summary by Davidson.[4] Twelve studies published since 1980 that focus on employment status following CABGS are summarized in Table 1 (pages 136-137).

These findings come from a wide range of geographic areas, sociocultural groups, and clinical settings in the United States and Canada. It is important to keep this diversity in mind when considering the variability of the data.

As indicated in Table 1, there is a 12-year span represented in this survey; the earliest patient population had surgery in 1968[10] and the most recent in 1980.[1] During this time, surgical techniques improved,[15] post-surgical hospital care changed, rehabilitation programs became more common, media attention to CABGS increased, and the number of annual CABGS procedures increased to approximately 170,000 in 1982.[16] Given these trends, it is likely that compared with 10 years ago, a current cardiac patient has a much higher likelihood of having known someone who had successful CABGS.

Length of post-surgical follow-up in these studies varied from 6 months[1] to 10 years,[10] most often being 1 to 2 years. Patient populations examined were mostly white men, although Guttman and co-workers[8] presented results for a small cohort of women. A meaningful comparison can be made between the employment statistics for cardiac patients and national labor statistics for similar groups of men of the same age distribution. In Johnson and colleagues'[10] 10-year follow-up, 2,812 men undergoing CABGS were investigated; the data were compared with national statistical averages during the 1970s. General employment trends during the time period of the study were as follows: employment rate was high (96-98%) for white men 40 years or older but dropped off rapidly after age 50. During the 1970s, there was an increased migration from the work force at age 50 and older, which was attributed to early voluntary retirement.[10]

For the employment statistics given in Table 1, working before surgery is denoted by "B" and working after surgery by "A." Not working before or after surgery are labeled $\overline{B}$ and $\overline{A}$, respectively. The four possible patterns of work before and after can then be denoted by: BA, B$\overline{A}$, $\overline{B}$A, $\overline{BA}$. It can be seen that there is wide variation in the percent working before surgery, (%B), varying from 47.9%, observed in the Jensen and associates'[9] study, to 91%, reported by Anderson and co-workers.[5] Whereas a low pre-surgical employment rate (50%) was also observed by Niles and associates,[13] all other values fall between 60% and 81%. This broad range is at least partly due to variation in age; for example, Stanton and colleagues[1] report a low pre-employment rate (41%) for patients at least 60 years of age. Other sources of variability are the social, cultural, and economic characteristics of the populations studied, and whether they are drawn from urban or rural geographic regions. The percent working at follow-up (%A) varied from 53% in the 1975-1977 study by Oberman and co-workers[2] to a high of 84% in the study by Jensen and associates.[9]

Probably the most important findings concern return to work after surgery (%BA). For patients less than 60 years old, these values range from 66% to 95%. Anderson and associates[5] found that patients were more likely to be working 1 year after surgery (72%) than they would be 3 years later (44%), although it is not clear whether this difference could be attributed to normal attrition that is related to retirement.

Results for individuals working before CABGS, but not after (B$\overline{A}$), representing percent disabled, present a mixed pattern; one study reported 17% disability[13] and another 5%.[9] The reasons patients give for not returning to work in these studies are as follows: Both Stanton and co-workers[1] and Johnson and colleagues[10] found that 53% of their patients tended to cite physical disability, whereas a few others cited "doctor's advice," and older patients often cited a "desire to relax." In the former study,[1] 24% of those who did not return to work found their time more enjoyable than expected, while 43% found it less pleasant. In a study of 949 patients who had recovered from CABGS, Zyzanski and associates[17] found the most negative emotional reactions among patients who had been working before surgery and were then forced to retire. The authors point out that forced retirement can lead to a loss of self-esteem and self-acceptance, and interfere with emotional adjustment in persons for whom an occupational role is central to self-concept. Similarly, Guttman and co-authors[8] found that B$\overline{A}$ "patients were significantly more distressed by weakness, fatigue, and physical limitations than the other three work status

TABLE 1: EMPLOYMENT STATUS

Authors, Study Period(s)	Follow-Up	Age (years)	Employment Statistics* %B	%A	%BA	%BA̅	%BA̅	%BA̅
Anderson et al[5]** 1969-1974	1-4 years	<55	95.9***	--	92.1***** 90.1	--	23.1***** 38.5	--
		55-59	92.9***	--	86.2***** 67.7	--	20.0***** 30.0	--
		>60	74.0***	--	71.6**** 44.4	--	17.9***** 10.7	--
		M̲	91	81***** 72	--	--	--	--
Boulay et al[6] 1969-1972	30 months	52.7	62	58	69	--	--	--
1973-1980	12 months	49.8	84	66	76	--	--	--
1978-1980	12 months	50.7	--	82	89	--	--	--
Gundle et al[7] 1976-1977	12-24 months	51.4	--	--	--	--	--	--
Guttman et al[8]** 1978-1979	12.5 months (avg)	57.7	69 75	58 64	82 82	18 18	7 10	93 90
Jensen et al[9]	1 year	<55 55-65	-- --	-- --	91.5 77.5	-- --	-- --	-- --
		M̲	47.9	84.2	95.4	4.6	74	26
Johnson et al[10]** 1968-1978	up to 10 years	--	78.8	79	87	13	50	50
Kornfeld et al[11] 1972-1975	up to 4-1/2 years	52.1	77	76***** 65	--	--	--	--

Authors, Study Period(s)	Follow-Up	Age (years)	Employment Statistics*					
			%B	%A	%BA	$\overline{\text{%BA}}$	$\overline{\text{%BA}}$	$\overline{\text{%BA}}$
Love[12] 1975-1977	15 months (avg)	55.6	64	54	70.5***	29.5***	23.5***	76.5***
Niles et al[13] 1976-1978	20 months	55.6	50	60	82.7	17.3	38***	62***
Oberman et al[2] 1970-1974	1 year	--	65	55	--	--	--	--
1975-1977	1 year	--	60	53	75	25	25	75
--	3 years	--	61.7	46.8	--	--	--	--
--	2 years	--	78.6	65	--	--	--	--
Smith et al[14]** 1974-1977	2 years	56.1	81	72	77	23	29	71
Stanton et al[1] 1979-1980	6 months	55	74.1		77.5	22.5	21.4	78.6
		55-59	68.9		74.5	25.5	21.7	78.3
		60-64	41.3		47.4	52.6	11.1	88.9
Average finding*****			67.9	66.3	76.6	23.1	27.6	69.9

* B denotes working before surgery, A denotes working after. Not working before or after are denoted by $\overline{\text{B}}$ and $\overline{\text{A}}$, respectively.
** All male patient population.
*** Our figures computed from authors' data.
**** Top figure = earlier follow-up; bottom figure = later follow-up.
***** Care should be taken in the interpretation of these figures due to variability among studies. All follow-up intervals included. Patient number varies from column to column.
M = group mean.

groups, which do not differ significantly from one another."

The proportion of individuals not working before surgery, but working at follow-up (%BA̅) varies, but usually is well under 50%. An exception is Jensen and colleagues' study,[9] which reports an employment gain of 74%. In the investigation by Anderson and associates[5] there was a greater gain in employment 4 years after surgery than at the 1-year follow-up in the patients less than 60 years old who were unemployed prior to surgery. A similar gain at 4 years is not found among those who were working before surgery. That more nonworking patients would increase employment after 4 years than previously working patients may illustrate a pattern discernible only with a longer follow-up.

Finally, a look at those patients not working before or after surgery (%B̅A̅) completes the picture. There is wide variability in this percentage: Guttman and co-workers[8] report 93%, whereas Jensen and associates[9] observed only 26%. However, most values were in the area of 70%.

EMPLOYMENT STATUS: PREDICTIVE VARIABLES

Table 2 (page 139) shows factors most commonly associated with employment status. Note that it has not been established whether or not they bear a causal relationship to employment; these associations are only correlational, and in many instances, statistical significance of these factors was not assessed. Where there is a high degree of association between a variable and employment, that variable can be understood to be a predictor of return to work, without making an assumption of causality. The variables are discussed in order of the frequency with which they were associated with employment.

PRE-SURGICAL EMPLOYMENT STATUS

Pre-surgical employment status was one of the preoperative variables most commonly associated with return to work. Patients who had worked before surgery were more likely to be employed following surgery. This finding was replicated in nearly every study surveyed for this chapter. In the study by Stanton and associates,[1] the answer to a single question, "Do you feel you will be able

TABLE 2: PREDICTIVE VARIABLES OF EMPLOYMENT STATUS

Authors	Pre-Surgical Employment Status	Age	Medical Status and Symptoms	Type of Occupation	Educational Level	Income	Other
Anderson et al[5] <55 years		+	+				MI in past; self-employed
≥55 years		+	+				Duration of symptoms
Boulay et al[6]	+	+	+	+	+		
Gundle et al[7]	+						
Guttman et al[8]		+	+	+		+	Disability compensation Graft patency not significant
Jensen et al[9]	+						
Johnson et al[10]		+					Physical disability; doctor's advice; desire to relax
Love[12]		+	+	+			
Niles et al[13]*	(1)	(5)	dyspnea (2) angina (3) fatigue (4)		(6)		Exercise tolerance test (7) Male sex (8)
Oberman et al[2]	+	+	+	+	+	+	Perception of health
Smith et al[14]**	(2)	(5)	angina (1) graft (6)	(4)			Post-op medication (3) CHF (7)
Stanton et al[1]*** Patients' expectations - .259			fatigue - .200 angina - .172		.184	.175	Trail-making test - .162 Use of religion - .137

* Ranked by size of effect in multivariate analysis.
** Ranked by size of effect in univariate analysis.
*** Values are multiple regression coefficients.
CHF = congestive heart failure; MI = myocardial infarction.

to go back to work after surgery?" was the most significant predictor of return to work. There are at least two important implications of this finding:

1. It may be possible to evaluate accurately the broad array of psychologic, biologic, and socioeconomic factors that influence return to work with a single question.
2. By and large, patients' expectations comprise an important mediating variable in employment plans. This is consistent with a large literature in psychology demonstrating that expectations and beliefs are major determinants of behavior.[18,19]

AGE

The biggest drop in post-surgical employment occurs after age 60.[1,5,9] However, employment rate falls off sharply in the general work force at this point as well. When CABGS patients are compared with age-matched reference groups in the general work force, the extent of relative disability actually diminishes with advancing age. In fact, patients 70 years and older had a higher employment rate than the general work force in one study.[10] The studies in which intragroup age comparisons were made yielded quite varied results.[1,5,9] However, these results, as well as reports by others,[12,20,21] are consistent with the general finding that employment rates of older CABGS patients can be expected to be lower than those of patients no more than 55 years old. From the diverse values observed, it is too early to estimate the relative size of this age-related discrepancy in employment.

The reasons for the age effect on employment rate are psychologic and sociologic, as well as medical. It is true that older patients are more likely to cite physical requirements of their work[5,22] and the reappearance of angina[5,23] as reasons for retirement. However, the reasons extend well beyond physical factors. The 60- to 70-year age range is the period in adult life when people most often retire. This psychologic landmark has been influenced by social pressure. Also, during the 1970s there was a trend toward earlier retirement.[10] Perhaps the study by Stanton and associates[1] reflects the earlier retirement expectations of this time period.

MEDICAL STATUS

Medical status before and after surgery was generally correlated with return to work following CABGS. Two variables that were consistently associated with retirement were angina and fatigue. Stanton and associates[1] found that the one pre-operative medical variable that predicted return to work was anginal class. Improvement in angina following surgery is associated with higher employment rates.[5,6,8,13,14] Two studies reported associations between post-operative fatigue and return to work,[8,13] whereas one found pre-operative fatigue (Profile of Mood States [POMS] fatigue score) to be the second best predictor (after patients' expectations concerning return to work) of employment after surgery.[1]

Attempts to examine more objective indicators of medical status, for example, number of diseased vessels, graft patency, and left ventricular ejection fraction (LVEF) have not yielded consistent findings. Niles and colleagues[13] and Roquebrune and associates[24] failed to confirm a correlation between the number of diseased vessels (often referred to as an index of severity of coronary artery disease) and return to work. These studies are not in agreement with the reported association found in earlier studies.[2,23] The results on graft patency are primarily derived from the study by Jensen and associates,[9] who did not find any significant relationship between graft patency and the overall percentage of patients working post-operatively. They did, however, observe a linear relationship between patency and work status when retirees and one-vessel graft recipients were excluded. These findings suggest that a relationship between graft patency and post-operative work status may hold only for certain subgroups of patients. In general, the authors conclude that factors other than graft patency and relief of symptoms may be responsible for post-operative work status. Smith and colleagues[14] report completeness of grafting as one of seven variables predictive of post-operative employment derived from a multivariate analysis, but do not suggest an explanation for these findings.

Guttman and co-authors[8] compiled LVEFs for the four work status groups and found them to be significantly higher in men in the BA group than in the other three groups. Niles and co-workers[13] and Johnson and colleagues[10] failed to confirm a significant relationship between ejection fraction and work status (except for severe impairment in the latter study). Other variables examined as factors related to work status have been post-operative medication (e.g., nitroglycerin[5] and propranolol[25]), post-operative exercise tolerance test,[13] and medical advice.[10]

Angina appears to be the most frequently reported medical symptom related to work status - its presence is directly correlated with a failure to return to work. The second most commonly identified symptom was fatigue. Patients whose fatigue was relieved by surgery had a higher post-operative employment rate. Results were less clear for the number of grafts, graft patency, LVEF, post-operative medication, and post-operative exercise tolerance test.

SOCIOECONOMIC VARIABLES

Occupational level, family income, and educational status are discussed together in this chapter because they are closely related. Educational level was found to be significantly positively correlated with employment in a number of studies.[1,4,13] According to Niles and associates,[13] it is not clear if this is attributable to a better understanding of the medical problem and treatment, greater job incentives, or to less physically demanding types of work. In the study by Stanton and co-workers,[1] education and family income were among the strongest independent predictors of return to work after surgery; both were stronger predictors than job type. In fact, educational level and family income eliminated the predictive contribution of occupational level and physical demands of the job.

Two other investigation teams found that physical activity as part of the patient's pre-operative occupation was an influential variable;[6,14] however, neither study examined family income. Another study cited occupational level as a determinant of return to work, but also found income to be significantly correlated with employment,[8] leaving open the possibility that the difference between work income and disability compensation was the important determinant. Physical exertion appears to be a significant independent factor in blue-collar workers[26] and in older patients.[5] The hypothesis suggested by these studies is that occupationally required physical exertion is expected to be highly correlated with a lower level of education and a lower level of family income; the latter two variables may be stronger predictors of return to work. The type of person most likely not to return to work was an individual in the middle or low socioeconomic class with respect to job, income, and educational levels and who was receiving disability compensation.[8]

A multiple factor model is necessary to understand work status, in much the same way that we use a multiple risk factor model to account for the incidence of coronary heart disease. Davidson's model[4] is perhaps the most comprehensive, listing eight major factors for determination of return to work: (a) medical; (b) psychologic; (c) sociodemographic, economic, and cultural; (d) individual work history and perceptions of prior work; (e) individual's perception of health and risk to life; (f) individual's perception of self; (g) influence and constraints of others; and (h) individual's expectations and predictions.

A second approach is to identify empirically specific biopsychosocial measures by multivariate ranking of the variables according to predictive importance. An example of such a table is presented by Stanton and colleagues[1] and shows the following variables in order of the magnitude of the standardized regression coefficient: (a) patient's pre-operative expectations, (b) POMS fatigue score, (c) presence of level 3 or 4 angina, (d) patient's education, (e) time to finish Trailmaking test part A, (f) family income, and (g) use of religion as moral support.

Perhaps it is too early to decide precisely which model is more useful in predicting a patient's return to work after CABGS or to estimate what share of the pie should be allotted to individual variables. However, there is a clear consensus that medical management is only one aspect of a complex process; the majority of influences on post-CABGS work status can be related to psychosocial variables. Psychosocial factors must be managed if the optimal work status decision for a particular individual is to be made.

PSYCHOLOGIC AND SOCIAL OUTCOMES OF CABGS

Although employment status following surgery is an important variable, meaningful dimensions of recovery can be measured by other indexes of psychologic and social function.

There are at least three different types of assessment approaches used in the studies reviewed in this article, and measurement in this area can be complex and difficult. One assessment technique is the subjective clinical impression of the investigator. A second technique is objective measurement based on questionnaires completed by the patient. In some studies using the latter approach, questionnaire items had been psychometrically assessed for reliability and validity, and standardized on appropriate populations, while in other studies these procedures were not followed. A third method of measurement used was either a semistructured or standardized interview. The most psychometrically adequate methods would seem to be the standardized ones (although the other techniques are useful for generating hypotheses). Discussion of measurement issues can be found in papers by Rahimtoola and co-workers[15] and Jenkins and colleagues.[26]

SOCIAL OUTCOMES

Social role function was explored with a questionnaire in the recovery study by Jenkins's group.[26] In most patients, reported household activities were unchanged from pre-surgical levels, although household chores showed some increase. Family dynamics were also examined, and one-half of the patients reported that the CABGS had brought their family closer together. There were also reports of overprotectiveness (36%), and about one-half of the patients believed that their family worried more about their health after the operation than before. Responses to three items concerning marital interaction were the same pre- and post-operatively in one-half to two-thirds of the patients.

Sexual activities and attitudes have received considerable attention.[27] Two investigative groups confirm a trend toward a less-active and less-satisfying sex life after surgery; another study does not. Kornfeld and colleagues[11] noted a drop in sexual activity 9 months after CABGS. Three and one-half years after surgery, sexual satisfaction decreased more and showed less improvement than five other measured attributes (i.e., pleasure, nervousness, mood, job satisfaction, and family relations). In the small cohort of patients studied by Gundle and associates,[6] sexual dysfunction was reported in 57% of the sample. Jenkins and colleagues,[26] however, found that 6 months after surgery, the level of sexual satisfaction was unchanged when compared with 1 year before surgery for one-half of their patients; it worsened in approximately 25% of this sample. (The change in sexual satisfaction was attributed by most patients to their energy level, that is, it either increased or decreased.) Weiss[28] has pointed out the importance of taking into account age, peer and cultural norms, and the prior sexual functioning level when evaluating sexuality in cardiac patients. The three studies cited above were within-subject comparisons and thus accurate assessment of pre-surgical sexual function would be especially important. For example, an individual's tendency to remember historical data inaccurately calls into question the validity of a comparison with the recalled frequency 1 year before surgery.

PSYCHOLOGIC OUTCOMES

The possibility that cognitive deficits may be an undesirable sequela of CABGS is of great interest. Jenkins and co-authors[26] and Savageau and associates[29] examined patients' psychoneurologic function using performance times on the Trailmaking A and B tests from the Halstead-Reitan Battery, visual reproduction scores on the Wechsler Memory Scale (WMS), and the Logical Memory subtest of the WMS.[26,30] Six months after surgery only 5% of the total group showed a decline from pre-operative levels. The Logical Memory subtest showed a statistically reliable increment. These findings support the inference that, on the average, CABGS is not associated with long-term adverse psychoneurologic effects. In fact, the data suggest the presence of some improvements in speed and concentration.

However, in a paper on unrecognized organic mental disorders in survivors of cardiac arrest, Reich and co-workers[30] point out the importance of passage of time in recognizing cerebral dysfunction. Subtle impairments such as fatigue, distractibility, and inability to learn new skills may be involved, as well as apathy and disturbances of judgment and insight. Information from family and friends who knew an individual well prior to surgery can facilitate diagnosis. Such variables are, of course, difficult to quantify and measure, but may, nevertheless, be important. Ramshaw and Stanley[31] found evidence pointing to the possibility of neurologic changes in the adaptive style observed in one subgroup of patients in their study of individual differences in lifestyle response to CABGS. They administered a battery of psychologic tests to 53 such patients and received patient self-reports. One subgroup of patients reported a higher than average incidence of memory problems as well as apparent personality changes. The authors speculate whether "subtle and persisting neurologic damage" may be associated with these changes.

Evidence that short-term cognitive deficits occur during the hospitalization period was also reported. Tirrell and Hart[32] found that approximately 25% of their subjects could not remember anything about their post-operative hospital stay and said they had found it hard to concentrate during the immediate post-operative period. This contributed to a number of knowledge-of-regimen deficits about the post-operative teaching program. Scalzi and colleagues[33] also found patients' retention of information during hospitalization to be limited. Instruction during the post-discharge period, with printed take-home material, appeared to facilitate the educational process and contributed to compliance in several areas. Aberg and co-authors[34] conclude that subclinical brain injury is often seen after cardiac operations, but the cause is unknown. Most often, the injury is reversible, but in a minority of cases, it is not.

Perhaps those psychologic outcomes that lend themselves more easily to direct measurement are the behavioral risk factors, for example, smoking, exercise, and weight. Kornfeld's group[11] found that smoking declined from 39% pre-operatively to 13% 9 months post-operatively; 38% of patients had changed their exercise pattern, but little change was observed in their weight. Compliance with cardiac medication was generally good (86% complied fully).

Type A behavior pattern is also an established coronary heart disease risk factor. Kornfeld and colleagues[11] found (a) a relatively large proportion of Type A individuals in their surgical sample (84%) and (b) the Type A pattern persisted in follow-up assessments. Nine months after surgery, 75% of patients were unchanged in regard to their rating; 7% had acquired more Type A characteristics, and 18% retained less. Decreases in characteristics often involved job commitment and time urgency. Severe angina also may have been correlated with a behavior change in individuals after a longer follow-up (3-1/2 years). Zyzanski and associates[17] assessed long-term recovery (average, 3 years) in 949 patients. Using a battery of scales, they found that Type A persons exhibited poorer social and emotional adjustment than Type B individuals, and reported more feelings of anxiety, depression, discouragement, and restlessness. Adjustment of the Type A person is also discussed by Gundle and co-workers.[6] In their study, involving a cohort of 30 patients, Type A individuals were more often employed, but were not better adapted overall or more sexually functional than other patients.

Examination of more subjective cognitive and emotional aspects of life after CABGS recently yielded a generally optimistic picture of improvement.[11,26] Jenkins and colleagues'[26] data were derived from 10 scales and an interview administered before and 6 months after surgery. Pre-operative questionnaire depression scores were low and dropped to very low levels post-operatively. Fatigue scores declined, degree of vigor scores rose, and the positive well-being scale also showed gains. Neither measures of self-esteem, sense of mastery, nor willingness to depend upon others were reportedly changed. Anxiety scores, as measured by the Spielberger Anxiety Scale, were higher on average than anxiety scores for a reference population of general medical and surgical patients. However, by 6 months post-surgery, the scores had dropped into the normal range, a change that is reported as significant, both clinically and statistically. In the study by Kornfeld's group,[11] results at 3-1/2 year follow-up indicated subjective improvement in pleasure in life and mood, and less nervousness. This contrasts with the authors' earlier findings[35] of considerable distress, social withdrawal, impaired sexual function, and impaired self-reliance in an interview at the 1-year follow-up.

In a 3-1/2 year follow-up study, three groups of patients with particularly poor psychosocial outcomes were identified.[17] As previously mentioned, significantly more negative social and emotional changes were found in previously working persons who were forced to retire after CABGS. A second category of poorly adjusting patients were women who had multiple bypasses, as compared with men who underwent CABGS or women who had cardiac valve surgery. The third predictor also correlated with a poor emotional and social outcome was the classification as Type A.

A small patient sample studied by Gundle and associates[6] generally exhibited poor psychologic and social outcomes. Self-report scales and an interview pre-operatively and 1 to 2 years post-operatively showed psychosocial impairments, such as a restricted and unpleasurable social life, low self-esteem, symptomatic depression, and serious distortions of body image. The socioeconomic status of this population may have been related to their poor recovery since over one-half were blue-collar workers. Those with limited education and income appeared to interpret the prolonged symptoms before surgery as meaning that they were "damaged." The formation of a damaged self-concept was associated with a reluctance to work and poor sexual function.

A question regarding accuracy in symptom reporting has been raised. If persons believe they have done all they can for their problem, for example, cardiac surgery, does that belief alter self-perceptions so that patients feel they have returned to normal? This changed perception might be expected to affect the way in which symptoms are detected, interpreted, and reported. Putting this another way, are post-CABGS patients less likely to confess symptoms?[36] Many of the variables employed to assess recovery are subjective, difficult to quantify objectively, and influenced by many factors, such as previous learning and expectations. Thus, symptom reports should be considered keeping in mind the individual's context and history. Patients' perceptions and beliefs concerning their health may be more important than clinical severity in determining feelings, functions, and plans for the future.[4,8]

DISCUSSION

Several comments may be made regarding return to work following surgery. When return to work decisions are made pre-operatively, 82% of patients who make positive predictions fulfill them. Those who give uncertain or negative responses appear considerably less likely to return to work.[1] These results raise questions concerning the information that patients used to make this early decision, and they also illustrate the critical role that expectations play in recovery following cardiac surgery. Evidence that recovery expectations and return to work may be unrealistically low is suggested in further work that found recovery experiences during the first 6 months post-operatively to be better than patients had anticipated, especially in terms of physical recovery.[26] About half of these patients did better, both physically and psychologically, than they expected, suggesting that some patients may make overly pessimistic predictions concerning their post-operative course. Methods for changing expectations, beliefs, and attitudes have been used effectively in several areas of psychology and are a special focus of intervention in cognitive and behavioral therapies.[37,38] These may be helpful adjuncts to treatment where prognostic signs for good medical recovery from surgery coexist with equivocal motivation for returning to work.

Another group found to make early pre-operative decisions of return to work are individuals with high pre-surgical levels of angina and fatigue.[1] One hypothesis concerning this result is that those suffering from these symptoms pre-operatively are being subjected to the type of uncontrollable, unpredictable, and painful stimuli that patients in conditioned helplessness experiments receive.[39,40] According to this research, when individuals repeatedly experience noxious, unpredictable events and perceive that their efforts to control these events are ineffective, they will adopt a passive, apathetic attitude, give up, and stop responding. Patients presenting with this history may have a lowered sense of self-efficacy as a result of their prior experiences and could be considered candidates for special intervention that is geared toward helping them reverse this learning. Therefore, one possibility that may forestall maladaptive work decisions is medical advice that patients delay any decision concerning return to work until they have had a chance to assess the effect of surgery. Special attention could be focused on correcting negative biases that patients may have developed by providing realistic information about symptom improvement, using role models or peer counseling, and encouraging them to try the "experiment" of returning to work in order to test themselves in the work situation before making a decision.

Current findings suggest that other individuals with a poor prognosis are those who were forced to retire.[8,17] These patients may be given special intervention to help them to deal with their sudden change in work status and to encourage the development of alternate activities and role definitions, preventing the loss of self-esteem that often accompanies forced retirement. Support groups may be especially helpful for these individuals.

Bypass Surgery: Psychologic and Social Outcomes

Review of the psychologic and social consequences of surgery indicates that high levels of anxiety commonly occur around the time of surgery, accompanied by cognitive deficits that make retention of information difficult. There is a drop in sexual activity in a moderate percentage of patients on long-term follow-up. In general, we have not found evidence to substantiate earlier reports of more serious problems, especially depression.[35,41-44] There may be several reasons for this.

One hypothesis is that improvements in surgical technique and changes in post-surgical care and treatment, for example, spending fewer days in intensive care units, have produced less emotional disruption. A second hypothesis is that more active participation in classes and rehabilitation programs soon after surgery is, first, a behavioral intervention effective in countering depression, consistent with cognitive-behavioral treatment approaches described by Beck and colleagues,[37] and second, a psychologic intervention having the advantages recommended by Mumford and associates.[44] Another possibility is that current research was not designed to collect follow-up data at times that the authors of the literature on myocardial infarction recovery suggest are critical for the onset of depression, for example, within a few days after the event or immediately following hospital discharge.[45-47] A fourth hypothesis is that existing instruments for the self-report of depression are insensitive to the type of depression observed following cardiac events, as reports of lower than normal levels of depression[26] in these patients do not seem consistent with clinical experience. A final hypothesis is that CABGS patients are, in fact, less likely to become depressed than their counterparts whose cardiac event is a myocardial infarction. Perhaps CABGS is a cardiac experience that differs in basic ways from having an infarction. For example, being given a choice to have surgery may help individuals feel more in control and therefore may moderate the emotional impact of this event.

More negative social and emotional reactions were experienced during recovery by persons classified as Type A individuals than by persons classified as Type B.[17] This suggests that Type A persons are more limited in their ability to cope with recovery from cardiac surgery than are Type B patients. There is also some evidence that Type A patients return to work faster than Type Bs.

Given the probability of poor psychosocial outcome among Type A individuals, however, this may be one instance where an early return to work is not a positive decision. More research would be useful to help answer the many questions raised about this subgroup of patients.

It is difficult to evaluate the quality of life for the approximately 34% of CABGS patients who retire following surgery - an estimated 57,000 individuals per year. Until this population is more extensively studied, the data obtained by Jenkins's group[26] may be used to furnish preliminary projections for how often the decision to retire worked out well. In their survey, approximately 24% did better than anticipated in retirement.[26] Thus, choosing not to return to work after surgery can be considered a good decision in about one-quarter of those patients who retire. This appears to be a promising area for future research.

Finally, the data summarized here suggest that relatively accurate predictions can be made regarding a return to work and other psychosocial outcomes after CABGS using a multivariate model. How this approach might be used in patient selection is unclear, but at least prospective evaluation of the pre-operative variables stressed here, relative to post-operative psychosocial outcome, is appropriate.

REFERENCES

1. Stanton BA, Jenkins CD, Denlinger P, Savageau JA, Weintraub RM, Goldstein RL: Predictors of employment status after cardiac surgery. *JAMA* 1983;249:907-911.
2. Oberman A, Wayne JB, Kouchoukos NT, Charles ED, Russell RO, Rogers WJ: Employment status after coronary artery bypass surgery. *Circulation* 1982;65(suppl 2):115-119.
3. Doehrman SR: Psycho-social aspects of recovery from coronary heart disease: A review. *Soc Sci Med* 1977;11:199-218.
4. Davidson DM: Return to work after cardiac events: A review. *J Cardiac Rehabil* 1983;3:60-69.
5. Anderson AJ, Barboriak JJ, Hoffman RG, Mullen DC: Retention or resumption of employment after aortocoronary bypass operations. *JAMA* 1980;243:543-545.
6. Boulay FM, David PP, Bourassa MG: Strategies for improving the work status of patients after coronary artery bypass surgery. *Circulation* 1982;66(suppl 3):43-49.

7. Gundle MJ, Reeves BR, Tate S, Raft D, McLaurin LP: Psychosocial outcome after coronary artery surgery. *Am J Psychiatry* 1980;137:1591-1594.
8. Guttman MC, Knapp DN, Pollock ML, Schmidt DH, Simon K, Walcott G: Coronary artery bypass patients and work status. *Circulation* 1982;66(suppl 2):33-42.
9. Jensen RL, Clayton PD, Liddle HV: Relationship between graft patency, post operative work status, and symptomatic relief. *J Thorac Cardiovasc Surg* 1982;83:503-511.
10. Johnson WD, Kayser KL, Pedraza PM, Shore RT: Employment patterns in males before and after myocardial revascularization surgery. *Circulation* 1982;65:1086-1093.
11. Kornfeld DS, Heller SS, Frank KA, Wilson SN, Malm JR: Psychological and behavioral responses after coronary artery bypass surgery. *Circulation* 1982;66(suppl 3):24-28.
12. Love JW: Employment status after coronary bypass operations and some cost considerations. *J Thorac Cardiovasc Surg* 1980;80:68-72.
13. Niles NW, Vander Salm TJ, Cutler BS: Return to work after coronary artery bypass operation. *J Thorac Cardiovasc Surg* 1980;79:916-921.
14. Smith HC, Hammes LN, Gupta S, Vlietstra RE, Elveback L: Employment status after coronary artery bypass surgery. *Circulation* 1982;65(suppl 2):120-125.
15. Rahimtoola SH, Grunkemeier GL, Teply JF, Lambert LE, Thomas DR, Sven YF, Starr A: Changes in coronary bypass surgery leading to improved survival. *JAMA* 1981;246:1912-1916.
16. Hold the eggs and butter. *Time* 1984; Mar 26:56-63.
17. Zyzanski SJ, Stanton BA, Jenkins CD, Klein MD: Medical and psychosocial outcomes in survivors of major heart surgery. *J Psychosom Res* 1981;23:213-221.
18. Kelly G: *The Psychology of Personal Constructs*. New York, Norton, 1955.
19. Bandura A: Self-efficacy: Toward a unifying theory of behavior change. *Psychol Rev* 1977;84:191-215.
20. Rimm AA, Barboriak JJ, Anderson AJ, Simon J: Changes in occupation after aorto coronary vein-bypass operation. *JAMA* 1976;236:361-363.
21. Geha AS, Baue AE: Early and late results of coronary revascularization with saphenous vein and internal mammary artery grafts. *Am J Surg* 1979;137:456-463.
22. Kushnir BA, Fox KM, Portal RW: Factors influencing the resumption of work, sexual activity and driving fol-

lowing acute myocardial infarction. *Am Heart J* 1977; 93:261-262.
23. Barnes GK, Ray AJ, Oberman A, Kouchoukos NT: Changes in working status of patients following coronary bypass surgery. *JAMA* 1977;238:1259-1262.
24. Roquebrune JP, Lienhard JF, Schmitt R, Bourlon F, Sabatier M, Kreitmann P: Preliminary study on the resumption of work after aortocoronary bypass. *Arch Mal Coeur* 1981;74:419-425.
25. Almeida D, Bradford JM, Wenger NK, King SB, Hurst JW: Return to work after coronary bypass surgery. *Circulation* 1983;68(suppl 2):209-213.
26. Jenkins CD, Stanton BA, Savageau JA, Denlinger P, Klein MD: Physical, psychological, social and economic outcomes six months after coronary artery bypass surgery. *JAMA* 1983;250:782-788.
27. Rahimtoola SH: Coronary bypass surgery for chronic angina - 1981. *Circulation* 1982;65:225-241.
28. Weiss T: What the physician needs to know about sex and the heart (commentary). *Medical Aspects of Human Sexuality* 1983;17:233-239.
29. Savageau JA, Stanton BA, Jenkins CD, Frater RWM: Neuropsychological dysfunction following elective cardiac operation. *J Thorac Cardiovasc Surg* 1982;84:595-600.
30. Reich P, Regestein QR, Murawski BJ, DeSilva RA, Lown B: Unrecognized organic mental disorders in survivors of cardiac arrest. *Am J Psychiatry* 1983;140:1194-1197.
31. Ramshaw JE, Stanley G: Individual differences in lifestyle response to coronary artery bypass surgery. *Br J Med Psychol* 1981;54:83-89.
32. Tirrell BE, Hart LK: The relationship of health beliefs and knowledge to exercise compliance in patients after coronary bypass. *Heart Lung* 1980;9:487-493.
33. Scalzi CC, Burke LE, Greenland S: Evaluation of an inpatient educational program for coronary patients and families. *Heart Lung* 1980;9:846-853.
34. Aberg T, Ronquist G, Tyden H, Brunnkvist S, Hultman J, Bergstrom K, Lilja A: Adverse effects on the brain in cardiac operations as assessed by biochemical, psychometric, and radiologic methods. *J Thorac Cardiovasc Surg* 1984;87:99-105.
35. Heller SS, Frank KA, Kornfeld DS, Malm JR, Bowman FO: Psychological outcome following open-heart surgery. *Arch Intern Med* 1974;134:908-914.

36. Kolata GB: Consensus on bypass surgery. *Science* 1981;211:43-44.
37. Beck AT, Rush AJ, Shaw BF, Emery G: *Cognitive Therapy of Depression.* New York, Guilford Press, 1979.
38. Burns D: *Feeling Good.* New York, William Morrow, 1980.
39. Seligman MET: *Helplessness: On Depression, Development, and Death.* San Francisco, Freeman, 1975.
40. Abramson LY, Seligman MET, Teasdale J: Learned helplessness in humans: Critique and reformulation. *J Abnorm Psychol* 1978;87:49-74.
41. Blacher RS: Paradoxical depression after heart surgery: A form of survivor syndrome. *Psychoanal Q* 1978;47:267-283.
42. Kimball CP: The experience of open heart surgery. *Arch Gen Psychiatry* 1972;27:57-63.
43. Rabiner CJ, Willner AE: Psychopathology observed on follow-up after coronary bypass surgery. *J Nerv Ment Dis* 1976;163:295-301.
44. Mumford E, Schlesinger HJ, Glass GV: The effects of psychological intervention on recovery from surgery and heart attacks: An analysis of the literature. *Am J Public Health* 1982;72:141-147.
45. Cassem NH, Hackett TP: Psychiatric consultation in a coronary care unit. *Ann Intern Med* 1971;75:9-14.
46. Wishnie HA, Hackett TP, Cassem NH: Psychological hazards of convalescence following myocardial infarction. *JAMA* 1971;215:1292-1296.
47. Razin AM: Psychosocial intervention in coronary artery disease. *Psychosom Med* 1982;44:363-387.

10

Organizational and Administrative Overview of Cardiac Rehabilitation Programs

Paul M. Ribisl

INTRODUCTION

The major focus of the other chapters in this volume is the psychosocial component of cardiac rehabilitation. Other forms of treatment that typically comprise a multidisciplinary approach to the rehabilitation of the patient with coronary heart disease (CHD) will be reviewed in this chapter. For practical reasons, this chapter will not provide a complete discussion of all areas, but rather will provide an overview of cardiac rehabilitation with ample reference to appropriate documents in the extant literature for the interested reader.

The incidence of CHD in the United States, after relatively low levels at the turn of the century, reached epidemic proportions in the mid to late 1960s. Since then, it has shown a dramatic decline of approximately 2-3% per year.[1] Nevertheless, it is the leading cause of death, accounting for more than 50% of the mortality from all causes. Epidemiologic studies, such as the Framingham Study,[2] have demonstrated that CHD has a multiple etiology that is related to an individual's inherited characteristics and lifestyle patterns which facilitate the atherogenic process. The purpose of cardiac rehabilitation is to restore the individual to optimal levels of psychologic, physiologic, and vocational function by promoting preventive behaviors such as smoking cessation, dietary modification, stress management, and increased levels of appropriate physical activity.

Organizational and Administrative Overview

ORGANIZATIONAL ISSUES

To insure the success of a comprehensive program of cardiac rehabilitation, there are several organizational issues that must be considered and resolved prior to the program's initiation. For the past 10 years, the rehabilitative staff at Wake Forest University has been involved in the development of cardiac rehabilitation programs throughout the state of North Carolina. The interested reader is referred to a recent publication for a detailed description of our 10-year experience.[3] The following key issues need to be addressed:

1. *Program Initiation and Planning.* At the outset, a planning team should be identified that would be comprised of a nucleus of individuals with both interest and expertise in the multiple intervention approach to cardiac rehabilitation. This group would act as a steering committee to provide guidance and structure to the program and would contain key individuals, including representative medical personnel, who are in a position to influence the development of the program within that community.
2. *Identification of Patient Potential.* A major problem facing many developing programs is the lack of an adequate referral base. For obvious economic reasons, this is a crucial factor in the success of any program and it requires an accurate and thorough appraisal of the potential sources of patient referrals. In our experience, an approach should include a *hospital survey*, a *physician survey*, and *contact with appropriate agencies* such as Vocational Rehabilitation. The hospital survey should be conducted to determine the number of patients within the community who are admitted annually for cardiovascular-related problems such as myocardial infarction, angina pectoris, and coronary artery bypass graft (CABG) surgery. The survey may generate unrealistic numbers since every potential patient is being counted. Of these potential patients, the physician survey should provide an estimate of the referrals that are likely to be made by community physicians, most likely cardiologists and internists. It has also been our experience that

less than a third of the estimated physician referrals are actually made in the year following the survey and this must be taken into account in the financial planning of the program.
3. *Medical Community Rapport.* Regardless of the magnitude of the patient potential, actual referrals are vitally linked to the cooperation of the community physicians. Therefore, early establishment of rapport with the medical community is essential. A successful approach we have used is to arrange an informational session at the County Medical Society in order to describe the nature of the program with the medical community. At this point, as well as in the initial physician survey, two points must be emphasized: first, that the program is both safe and effective and second, that the program is an *extension* of the physician's own care and medical supervision of their patient - *it is not a replacement.* In addition, printed materials should be developed, in the form of brochures or pamphlets, which describe the program and explain the procedures for application and admission.
4. *Personnel Required in a Cardiac Rehabilitation Program.* Another important characteristic of a successful program is the assembly of an enthusiastic, qualified, and capable staff. While all members of the team are important, two central figures (medical director and program director) should be identified early. The *program director*, who is responsible for the organizational and administrative aspects of the program, recruits and coordinates the efforts of the rest of the team and the success of the program is largely dependent on how well these duties are executed. On the other hand, the *medical director* is the primary link to the medical community and the rate of referrals to the program is dependent upon his/her rapport with other community physicians. The medical director must be well-respected by the referral physicians and should not represent a threat with regard to losing patients from their practice to the medical director or other physicians associated with the program.

Other personnel who comprise the multidisciplinary team include an *exercise specialist*, a *nutritionist/dietitian*, a *psychologist*, a *vocational counse-*

Organizational and Administrative Overview

lor, and a *business manager/secretary*. In most circumstances, budgetary restraints limit many of the personnel to a part-time employment status. Whenever possible, personnel should be licensed or certified; this issue is discussed at the end of this chapter.

5. *Facilities and Equipment.* The nature of the facilities and equipment will necessarily depend upon the size and the scope of the program, but certain considerations are important. The facility should be in a convenient and accessible location for the staff and participants, since this is one of the major factors affecting initial and continuing participation in a program. The facility should satisfy the present as well as future size and availability needs of the program. The facilities and equipment should accommodate the multiple intervention approach, including the assessment, prescriptive, and therapeutic phases of each discipline (medical, exercise, dietary, psychologic, and vocational). Concurrently, the rental/overhead expenses should be reasonable so as not to jeopardize the affordability of the program. Specific guidelines regarding minimal standards for both facilities and equipment are described elsewhere.[4]

6. *Finance and Budget.* While success of a program is dependent upon many factors, even the best programs cannot survive without adequate financial support. In the planning stages, it is essential that sufficient funds be identified to support the program for the initial months in which income does not offset expenses. The source of these initial funds may include grants, seed money, and corporate and/or personal donations; it is important to realize that the starting date of the program should be delayed until at least 3 to 6 months of expenses can be covered, since that is the usual delay in generating revenues from the two major sources - insurance carriers and patient fees.

No program can operate without the revenues from third-party carriers since patients are rarely capable of covering the total cost of a program. Patient fees are typically used only to cover the balance remaining after the insurance payment. Therefore, it is suggested that the appropriate members of the steering committee meet with the professional representatives of those insurance companies that will most likely cover the highest percentage of patients in the program. At this time, the level of reimbursement for the services provided by the program can be determined and important details can be settled, such as obtaining a provider number, an employer ID number, and tax-exempt status. In addition, recommended procedures for filing claims can be established. Failure to secure adequate third-party coverage, in most cases, will seriously jeopardize the financial status of the program.

PROGRAM ISSUES

While the previous section dealt with the planning and preparatory stages of developing a program, the following section will cover the essential components of a multiple intervention program. Several recent publications may be consulted for a more detailed treatment of this topic.[5,6,7,8,9]

PATIENT ADMISSION CRITERIA

Specific admission criteria for potential patients must be established prior to the initiation of the program since these criteria will dictate the composition of the patient population and the nature of the program being developed. These criteria should be communicated to the medical community so that appropriate referrals will take place; the criteria can also be used to classify patients for eligibility for third-party reimbursement of patient services. Common criteria include:

1. Myocardial infarction
2. Angina pectoris
3. Post-operative cardiovascular surgery (CABG, angioplasty, valve repair or replacement)
4. Other diagnoses including patients with cardiovascular related disorders such as arrhythmias, pacemakers, hypertension, or other conditions requiring special attention
5. In recent years, patients with chronic obstructive pulmonary disease, renal disease, and diabetes are frequently included since these disorders may be associated with cardiovascular dysfunction

Organizational and Administrative Overview

Prior to admission to the program it is recommended that all patients be referred by their physician (family physician and/or specialist) and that the referral be accompanied by a medical history, discharge summary, and diagnosis.

ASSESSMENT, PRESCRIPTION, THERAPY, AND FOLLOW-UP

The multiple intervention approach to rehabilitation of the patient with CHD is comprised of four distinct, but inter-related, steps that include *assessment*, *prescription*, *therapy*, and *follow-up* in the following areas: medical/laboratory, exercise, nutritional, psychologic, and vocational. The assessment and prescription are made upon entry to the program and are basis for the therapy, while follow-up is made at regular intervals, usually at 3, 6, and 12 months after entry.

Medical/Laboratory. The *assessment* in the medical/laboratory phase is made after a careful review of the patient's medical history including disease diagnosis, medications, and discharge summary. For a more detailed description of the medical aspects of this assessment, the interested reader is referred to the guidelines prepared by the American College of Sports Medicine.[10] The medical director is responsible for this review and should make the determination that there are no contraindications to either exercise testing or training for the patient. The assessment should include a physical examination that evaluates the presence of any acute illness, orthopedic problems, and noncardiovascular problems, as well as a brief cardiovascular evaluation using auscultation and palpation procedures to detect significant abnormalities. The laboratory tests should include measures of body composition, and an assessment of risk factors for CHD: family history, smoking habits, serum lipids including the total cholesterol and high density lipoprotein (HDL) ratio, triglycerides and serum glucose, resting electrocardiogram (ECG) and blood pressure, and pulmonary function.

The information obtained from the medical/laboratory evaluation may be used to develop a specific *prescription* for medical *therapy* and/or further testing. However, the medical director normally uses this information to provide information and direction to the other members of the team during the subsequent patient staffing meeting.

Organizational and Administrative Overview

Follow-up is made at regular intervals unless dictated by unusual signs and symptoms.

Exercise. The primary approach used in the exercise *assessment* is the graded exercise test (GXT). This test is supplemented with additional information such as determination of body composition, pulmonary function, and orthopedic status. Extensive treatment of the topic of graded exercise testing can be found elsewhere.[10,11,12,13,14]

After reviewing the medical information and obtaining an informed consent, the exercise testing *mode* (e.g., treadmill, bicycle, or arm ergometer) and *protocol* should be determined. The mode is determined on the basis of the type of training to be recommended. Patients who have no orthopedic problems will usually enter a walk/jog program; thus, the treadmill is the mode of choice. For those with orthopedic or peripheral vascular problems such as intermittent claudication, either the bicycle or arm ergometer would be more appropriate. While many different testing protocols exist, certain principles apply. Specifically, the test should begin at a low level (2-3 METs* for most cardiac patients) and increase gradually in intensity (1 MET/stage with 2-3 min stages) until volitional fatigue or signs/symptoms of exertional intolerance. While under the supervision of a physician, the following measures should be monitored continuously throughout the graded exercise test: ECG and heart rate, blood pressure, patient appearance, rating of perceived exertion (RPE), and patient signs and symptoms of angina pectoris and dyspnea. The criteria for test termination include abnormal changes in the ECG (ischemia-induced ST segment depression, frequent and/or dangerous dysrhythmias, blocks, etc.), inappropriate chronotropic or inotropic response (heart rate, blood pressure, and rate pressure product), and other signs of exertional intolerance. Upon completion of the graded exercise test, the results are then summarized and interpreted by the attending physician to be used in the subsequent prescription.

The exercise *prescription* and *therapy* is based upon the results of the graded exercise test. This topic is treated extensively in the aforementioned references and a special two-part issue on exercise prescription.[15] Generally, each exercise session is usually composed of a warm-up

---

*1 MET = 3.5 ml O_2/kg/min or the equivalent of resting metabolic rate.

phase, an aerobic stimulus phase, and a cool-down phase. During warm-up, range-of-motion and stretching exercises are used along with mild aerobic exercise. The major components of an exercise prescription include the *intensity*, *duration*, and *frequency* applied to a specific *mode* of exercise. The aerobic stimulus phase is usually performed through a walk/jog, leg and/or arm cycling, or swimming mode of exercise. The *intensity* is prescribed at a safe level of intensity on the basis of the results of the graded exercise test and is usually set at an intensity between 60-85% of the patient's symptom-limited functional capacity. Intensity is usually controlled through monitoring heart rate, ECG, and signs and symptoms (RPE, angina pectoris, dyspnea, etc.) throughout the exercise session. The *duration* of exercise is dependent upon the intensity; however, it is usually 30 to 45 minutes at an intensity of 60-85% of capacity, after the initial adjustment phase. The recommended *frequency* is usually alternate days or 3 to 4 days per week, at the optimal intensity and duration.

In addition to the warm-up, aerobic stimulus phase, and cool-down, the exercise *therapy* should adhere to the principles of overload, progression, and specificity. A starter program should precede the overload phase and is used to insure the safe and effective adaptation of the individual to the exercise prescription as well as prevent orthopedic and cardiovascular complications of exercise. The overload should be achieved through gradual increases in the energy demand during the stimulus phase resulting from a progressive increase in intensity and/or duration to optimal levels.

Short-term *follow-up* is made daily by recording intensity, duration, and frequency of exercise as well as noting signs/symptoms during the exercise sessions. Long-term follow-up occurs during repeat evaluations of functional capacity.

Nutritional. The primary objective of the nutritional component is the reduction of nutrition-related coronary risk factors (hyperlipidemia, obesity, hyperglycemia, and hypertension) through modification of the patient's diet and eating behavior. For a more detailed coverage of this topic, the reader is referred to other publications,[16,17,18,19] and to Chapter 1 in this volume. Only basic principles and methods are covered here.

Organizational and Administrative Overview

The nutritional *assessment* on entry into the program should be complete. For example, the Wake Forest Program includes:

- *Nutritional history* of past eating behavior, including any prescribed therapeutic diet, the use of sugar, salt, and alcohol;
- *Seven-day diary* of everything the patient eats and drinks and how the food is prepared;
- *Related information* including serum lipids (total cholesterol [TC], HDL, TC/HDL ratio, and triglycerides), serum glucose, height, weight, percent body fat, and current medications. Additional information from the patient's medical file regarding history of heart disease, hypertension, diabetes, and other related problems should be considered.

The above information is analyzed to determine the patient's needs. The analysis should determine if nutrition is adequate in terms of the total calories, essential foods and nutrients, fat content, and sodium intake. In addition, a determination should be made of ideal body weight based on anthropometric data and the desirable serum lipid levels relative to the patient's medical status.

The dietary *prescription* for each patient is based upon the above diagnosis and should be designed to achieve an ideal weight goal, a recommended caloric intake, optimal nutritional intake of all essential foods (Carbohydrate - 55%, Fat - 30%, and Protein - 15%), moderation of alcohol, caffeine and empty calorie consumption, adequate fiber intake, and control of sodium and saturated fat consumption. The implementation of this prescription should conform to any current diet prescription by the patient's physician.

Dietary *therapy* should consist primarily of a consultation with the patient and spouse to discuss new or existing diet orders and to recommend procedures for the implementation of the diet (e.g., exchange lists). During the consultation, food models, food packages, measuring cups, and spoons can be used to aid in the education of the patient and spouse regarding proper food preparation and basic shopping. Posters, booklets, flip charts, or slide-tape presentations are supplementary alternatives. It should be pointed out that the goal of the therapy is to assist the patient in making *permanent* rather than *short-term* modifications in eating habits and behavior. Behavior modification classes have also been shown to be effective.[20]

After the therapeutic sessions, continued *follow-up* is necessary to monitor progress toward the dietary and weight goals. Weekly weight checks are useful, while repeat measures of skinfold, girth measurements, serum lipid levels, and dietary intake should be conducted at routine intervals (3, 6, and 12 months).

Psychological. It was mentioned previously that little emphasis in this chapter would be placed on the psychosocial aspects of cardiac rehabilitation, since the assessment and treatment are reviewed in Chapters 2-9. Nevertheless, a brief overview of the topic will be presented as it relates to the approach used in our rehabilitative program at Wake Forest.[21]

The *assessment* phase should take into consideration the major concerns in dealing with the cardiac patient, including the nature of the stressors in the individual's life, the mechanisms of coping, their control beliefs, social relations, and lifestyle management. An assessment of these concerns can be made through:

- *Psychometric measures* include personality inventories (MMPI, 16PF, CPI), tests of anxiety (Spielberger's STAI), depression (Zung), or Type-A behavior (Jenkins Activity Survey). More recently, other instruments have been gaining in popularity since they have been designed with the medical population in mind; these include the Millon Behavioral Health Inventory, the SCL-90 test,[22] and a self-report measure of Type A behavior.[23] (See also, Chapter 2.)
- *Psychophysiological testing* in which heart rate, blood pressure, and/or other measures are monitored at baseline, after exposure to a mild stressor and in recovery to assess the individual's physiologic response to psychological stress.
- *Interviews* can also be useful, especially if they are structured and address the previously identified concerns (Rejeski, 1986).

The *prescription* will be based upon the recommendations derived from a careful analysis of the assessment data and can be administered in the form of psychotherapy (individual, group, or family), stress management, goals for re-establishing an appropriate level of psychosocial functioning, and guidelines for patient management.

While major forms of psychological dysfunction may be identified and require attention, these may be referred to specialists outside the cardiac rehabilitation program. The *therapy* most commonly utilized in the cardiac rehabilitation setting is related to the modification of health behaviors such as stress management, smoking cessation, and compliance with the exercise and nutritional recommendations. These are not as easily influenced by traditional forms of psychotherapy; it may be more practical and effective to utilize a multimodal cognitive/behavioral approach that involves self-monitoring in conjunction with motivation, stimulus control, cognition, and consequences of behavior.

Follow-up of the progress of patients towards the established goals can be done through daily contact with patients by program personnel, spot checks by the psychologist during the daily exercise sessions, and repeat testing with convenient, easily administered and scored instruments, such as the SCL-90.

Vocational. Ischemic heart disease is a leading cause of occupational disability in this country, and return to work is of major concern to many patients after a coronary event. While studies indicate that nearly 80% of previously employed patients do return to work, some of these patients fail to remain employed for the long term. For a more thorough treatment of vocational assessment and prescription, the interested reader is referred to the work of Sheldahl and others.[24]

The purpose of occupational *assessment* procedures is to determine if it is feasible for patients to return to work on the basis of their capacity for the demands of the job and to identify modifiable problems which may act as a deterrent to return to work. The vocational counselor should utilize the information already available from the assessments made by other team members (medical/laboratory, exercise, nutritional, and psychologic) since this information can provide insights about vocational rehabilitation. The assessment should include the following:

- *Clinical assessment* should include the pertinent data from the medical history, such as disease

Organizational and Administrative Overview

diagnosis and cardiac-related tests (physical exam, catheterization, echocardiography, nuclear imaging, etc.), to provide insight into the cardiovascular status of the patient.
- *Job demands assessment* can be accomplished through a questionnaire, an interview, and/or on-site inspection of the working conditions. The important factors to be assessed include the type of work (static/dynamic), the energy demands (light/heavy), environmental stress (heat/pollution/noise), and psychologic stress.
- *Functional capacity testing* will provide an estimate of the patient's ability to meet the physical demands of the work.
- *Simulated work testing* will provide a measure of the patient's capacity for the demands related to a specific job.

The *prescription* and *therapy* recommended for each patient will necessarily depend upon the results of the assessment. If the assessment reveals medical problems, an appropriate solution may be medication or surgery. If the physical job demands are beyond the patient's capacity, exercise training (strength and/or aerobic training) may be appropriate. If the demands are environmental or psychological, then modification of the approach to the job may be useful. If the demands are beyond the realistic changes which can be brought about through medical management, exercise training, or job modification, it is likely that vocational retraining may be the only viable alternative.

The *follow-up* can be accomplished by routine contacts at the time of their routine retesting with the patients who are employed, usually at 3, 6, and 12 months.

TEAM APPROACH AND PATIENT STAFFING PROCEDURES

The team approach is essential if the multiple intervention strategy is to be utilized effectively. At the end of the assessment phase, when each of the staff members has made a careful and thorough assessment of each patient, the team should assemble to discuss each case and share the results of their evaluation. The expertise provided by each team member on the case may alter the prescriptive and therapeutic recommendations of one or

Organizational and Administrative Overview

more team members or merely reinforce their decisions. At the end of the discussion, a summary should be prepared, in the form of a written report, which reflects the assessment and prescription developed by each team member.

REPORTS TO REFERRAL PHYSICIANS/PROGRESS NOTES

In order to maintain contact and rapport with the medical community, the staffing report prepared by the team should be shared with the referral physician(s). In addition, the goals for each patient should be shared with staff members who interact with patients daily so that they may be supportive of the patient's efforts toward achieving these goals.

Patient Education. Patient education is a vital component of any cardiac rehabilitation program and can provide complementary support to the intervention strategies of all disciplines. While knowledge and understanding do not automatically infer compliance, in many cases they can provide the incentive and motivation necessary for behavior change. For a more detailed discussion of the topic of patient education, the interested reader is referred elsewhere.[25,26] The Wake Forest program includes a review of the following areas:

- *Goals and Objectives.* The goals and objectives may differ among the different phases of cardiac rehabilitation and this should be considered in the development of an educational program. For instance, the in-hospital program stresses the responsibility of self-care and attempts to educate the patient in a broad spectrum of knowledge and responsibilities (nature of the disease, knowledge of risk factors, understanding of medications, and recognition of warning signs and symptoms). The early out-patient program primarily reinforces previous concepts and supports their practical application to daily living, while the community out-patient program may attempt to maintain positive changes in lifestyle and foster a lifetime commitment to health maintenance.
- *Program.* Before the program can be developed, certain issues should be resolved. Since few pro-

grams can afford a specialist in patient education, one individual should be assigned to conduct the educational intervention program. This individual will be responsible for determining the nature of the educational program, including the type of intervention, the frequency of sessions, the materials to be used, and the type of reinforcement.
- *Methods.* In order to meet the educational objectives of a program, several factors should be considered. These include: (a) establishment of good rapport between the staff and the patient, (b) assessment of the level of patient knowledge at entry, (c) establishment of a plan to meet individual educational needs, (d) provision for alternative information sources where appropriate, and (e) evaluation to determine whether the goals have been achieved.

EMERGENCY PROCEDURES

Due to the nature of the population being served, perhaps one of the most important components of a cardiac rehabilitation program is the development of an effective procedure to handle medical emergencies. Thompson[27] indicates that the cardiovascular risk of cardiac rehabilitation has been quantified, being placed at one episode of cardiac arrest and one death for every 33,000 and 120,000 patient hours of exercise, respectively. This suggests that the risk of exercise does not exceed the benefits. While the risk of an event may be low, the ability of the staff to handle an event properly can markedly reduce the mortality rate associated with a program in spite of having high-risk patients. This topic is covered in more detail elsewhere,[28] but the basic essentials of an emergency program include the following:

1. *Staff Qualifications and Training.* All personnel associated with the program should be certified in Basic Life Support (American Heart Association, American Red Cross) with at least one staff member certified in Advanced Cardiac Life Support.
2. *Emergency Plan.* A formal, written emergency plan should be developed which is specific to each program and should include the entire facility utilized by the program (gyms, laboratories, lockers/showers, offices). This plan should follow

standard/accepted procedures for the immediate stabilization of the patient and transfer to a medical facility, and also include the staff assignments, emergency equipment, supplies, and drugs required.
3. *Staff Emergency Assignments.* At the start of each exercise session, each staff member should be assigned a specific role to fulfill in the event of an emergency. This will serve to remind each staff member of his/her responsibilities and insure that all roles are covered each day.
4. *Emergency Procedures.* A detailed description of the roles and duties of each staff member should be described in the written emergency plan. Emergency drills should be practiced until there are no significant problems and then repeated at least monthly thereafter. Records of each drill should be maintained for review and potential liability inquiries.
5. *Equipment, Supplies, and Drugs.* A complete set of *equipment* (defibrillator, airways/intubation, oxygen tank and mask, ambu bag, suction, etc.), *supplies* (intravenous sets, syringes, needles, tape, etc.), and *drugs* (sodium bicarbonate, epinephrine, lidocaine, nitroglycerin, atropine, etc.) should be maintained in proper working order and supply.

CERTIFICATION OF PROGRAMS AND PERSONNEL

The field of cardiac rehabilitation is relatively new in relationship to other fields; therefore, licensure and certification within rehabilitation is limited primarily to certain personnel rather than to the programs themselves. This section will discuss the present status of the certification of programs and personnel in cardiac rehabilitation.

NATIONAL STANDARDS

The basis for the development of certification programs is the existence of current standards, policies, and procedures which govern the operations within a specialty area. Currently, two standards exist which should be used for guidance in establishing certification within cardiac rehabilitation: The American College of Sports Medicine's guidelines for exercise testing and prescription[10] and the American Heart Association's standards for exercise

Organizational and Administrative Overview

testing equipment, exercise testing laboratories, and exercise treatment programs.[29,30,31,32] These standards would also form the basis for any litigation involving exercise testing and/or training in cardiac rehabilitation programs.[33]

NORTH CAROLINA CARDIAC REHABILITATION ASSOCIATION (NCCR)

Approximately 6 years ago, a group of individuals from the numerous cardiac rehabilitation programs within the state of North Carolina formed an association to discuss issues related to cardiac rehabilitation. The association has elected officers, a board of directors, a constitution, and bylaws. There is an annual meeting with a formal program of invited speakers; in addition, several informal study groups within each of the disciplines meet to share information and discuss common problems. This association has been instrumental in the formulation of the guidelines for certification of programs of cardiac rehabilitation within the state, as described below.

NORTH CAROLINA RULES GOVERNING CARDIAC REHABILITATION PROGRAMS

In 1978 the NCCR Association adopted the NCCR Plan, a set of standards which served as guidelines for the certification of programs of cardiac rehabilitation within North Carolina. In 1983, a new standards document was ratified by the North Carolina General Assembly under GS Chapter 131E, Article 8, "Cardiac Rehabilitation Certification Program." These standards cover all aspects of a cardiac rehabilitation program (guidelines for personnel, facilities/equipment, programs, admission, assessment, prescription, therapy, follow-up, discharge, medical records, emergencies, and certification procedures) and are used by the Division of Facilities Services and the Division of Vocational Rehabilitation in the Department of Human Resources in the certification of programs of cardiac rehabilitation within North Carolina. The document is available from the Division of Vocational Rehabilitation Services (P.O. Box 26053, Raleigh, NC 27611). In addition to its value in providing a standard of care for patients in cardiac rehabilitation programs in North Carolina, the certificate is required by Blue

Cross/Blue Shield of North Carolina before a provider number can be issued and used in the request for reimbursement of cardiac rehabilitation services. The North Carolina Vocational Rehabilitation Agency likewise uses the certificate as a requirement for reimbursement. To our knowledge, this is the only state certification plan in existence that has been ratified by the state government and required by state insurance carriers and agencies. For a complete description of the certification process, see Graden.[34]

CERTIFICATION OF PERSONNEL BY THE AMERICAN COLLEGE OF SPORTS MEDICINE

Since 1975, the American College of Sports Medicine (ACSM) has been certifying personnel as preventive and rehabilitative program directors, exercise specialists, and exercise test technologists. These are individuals who are qualified to administer graded exercise tests; to execute exercise prescriptions; to design, supervise, and lead appropriate exercises; and to design, implement, and, administer safe, effective, and enjoyable preventive and rehabilitative exercise programs. A description of the behavioral objectives for each of these levels of certification can be found in ACSM.[10] For more information on certification contact: Director of Certification Programs, American College of Sports Medicine, P.O. Box 1440, Indianapolis, IN 46206. Certification workshops and certification sessions are offered throughout the nation several times each year.

REFERENCES

1. Dwyer T, Hetzel B: A comparison of trends of coronary heart disease mortality in Australia, USA and England and Wales with reference to 3 major risk factors - hypertension, cigarette smoking and diet. *Int J Epidem* 1980;9:65.
2. Kannel WB: Epidemiologic insights into atherosclerotic cardiovascular disease from the Framingham study, in Pollock ML, Schmidt DH (eds): *Heart Disease and Rehabilitation*. 2nd Ed. New York, John Wiley & Sons, 1986.

3. Miller HS, Ribisl PM, Adams GE, Boone WT, Morley D: Community programs of cardiac rehabilitation, in Pollock ML, Schmidt DH (eds): *Heart Disease and Rehabilitation.* 2nd Ed. New York, John Wiley & Sons, 1986.

4. North Carolina Department of Human Resources: *Rules Governing the Certification of Cardiac Rehabilitation Programs.* Division of Facility Services, 701 Barbour Drive, Raleigh, NC 27603.

5. Acierno LJ: *Comprehensive Cardiac Rehabilitation and Prevention: A Model Program.* New York, Immergut & Siolek Publishers, Inc., 1985.

6. Franklin BA, Rubenfire M (eds): Symposium on cardiac rehabilitation. *Clinics in Sports Medicine* 1984; 3(2):295-563.

7. Pollock ML, Schmidt DH (eds): *Heart Disease and Rehabilitation.* 2nd Ed. New York, John Wiley & Sons, 1986.

8. Wenger NK, Hellerstein HK (eds): *Rehabilitation of the Coronary Patient.* 2nd Ed. New York, John Wiley & Sons, 1984.

9. Wilson PK, Fardy P, Froelicher V: *Cardiac Rehabilitation, Adult Fitness and Exercise Testing.* Philadelphia, Lea & Febiger, 1981.

10. American College of Sports Medicine: *Guidelines for Exercise Testing and Prescription.* 3rd Ed. Philadelphia, Lea & Febiger, 1986.

11. Chung EK: *Exercise Electrocardiography: Practical Approach.* 2nd Ed. Baltimore, Williams & Wilkins, 1983.

12. Froelicher VF: *Exercise Testing and Training.* New York, Le Jacq Publishing, Inc., 1983.

13. Hellerstein HK, Franklin BA: Exercise testing and prescription, in Wenger NK, Hellerstein HK (eds): *Rehabilitation of the Coronary Patient.* 2nd Ed. New York, John Wiley & Sons, 1984.

14. Jones NL, Campbell EJM: *Clinical Exercise Testing.* 2nd Ed. Philadelphia, WB Saunders Company, 1982.

15. Pollock ML: Exercise prescription (Editorial). *J Cardiopulmon Rehabil* 1986;6(2&3):45-112.

16. Ellis J: Guidelines for nutritional evaluation and therapy, in Ribisl PM, et al: *Organizational Guidelines for Cardiac Rehabilitation Programs.* Winston-Salem, NC, Wake Forest Cardiac Rehabilitation Program, 1986.

17. American Heart Association: (Report of Nutrition Committee). Rationale of the diet-heart statement of the American Heart Association. *Circulation* 1982;65(4):839A-854A.

18. American Heart Association: (Joint statement of the Nutrition Committee and the Council on Arteriosclerosis). Recommendations for treatment of hyperlipidemia in adults. *Circulation* 1984;69(4):1065A-1090A.
19. *Heart to Heart: A Manual on Nutrition Counseling for the Reduction of Cardiovascular Disease Risk Factors*, NIH publication 80-1666. US Department of Health and Human Services.
20. Brownell KD: Obesity: Understanding and treating a serious, prevalent and refractory disorder. *J Consult Clin Psychol* 1982;50:820-840.
21. Rejeski WJ: Psychological care: assessment, prescription and therapy, in Ribisl PM, et al: *Organizational Guidelines for Cardiac Rehabilitation Programs*. Winston-Salem, NC, Wake Forest Cardiac Rehabilitation Program, 1986.
22. Derogatis LR: *SCL - 90(R) Manual - I*. Baltimore, The Johns Hopkins University School of Medicine, 1977.
23. Blumenthal JA, Herman S, O'Toole LC, Haney TL, Williams RB, Barefoot JC: Development of a brief self-report measure of the Type A (coronary prone) behavior pattern. *J Psychosom Res* 1985;265-274.
24. Sheldahl LM, Wilke NA, Tristani FE: Exercise prescription for return to work. *J Cardiopulmon Rehabil* 1985;5(12):567-575.
25. Morley D: Guidelines for patient and family education, in Ribisl PM, et al: *Organizational Guidelines for Cardiac Rehabilitation Programs*. Winston-Salem, NC, Wake Forest Cardiac Rehabilitation Program, 1986.
26. Bille DA: *Practical Approaches to Patient Teaching*. Boston, Little, Brown & Co., 1981.
27. Thompson PD: The cardiovascular risks of cardiac rehabilitation. *J Cardiopulmon Rehabil* 1985;5(7):321-324.
28. Morley D, Miller HS: Emergency procedures, in Ribisl PM, et al: *Organization Guidelines for Cardiac Rehabilitation Programs*. Winston-Salem, NC, Wake Forest Cardiac Rehabilitation Program, 1986.
29. American Heart Association: (Subcommittee on Rehabilitation Target Activity Group). Standards for Adult Exercise Testing Laboratories, publication 70-041-A. *Circulation* 1979;59:421A
30. American Heart Association: (Subcommittee on Rehabilitation Target Activity Group). Specifications for Exercise Testing Equipment, publication 70-041-A. *Circulation* 1979;59:849A.

31. American Heart Association: (Subcommittee on Rehabilitation Target Activity Group). Standards for Cardiovascular Exercise Treatment Programs, publication 70-041-A. *Circulation* 1979;59:1084A.

32. American Heart Association: (Subcommittee on Rehabilitation Target Activity Group). Standards for Supervised Cardiovascular Exercise Maintenance Programs, publication 70-041-A. *Circulation* 1980;62:669A.

33. Herbert DL, Herbert WG: *Legal Aspects of Preventive and Rehabilitative Exercise Programs.* Canton, OH, Professional and Executive Reports and Publications, 1985.

34. Graden H: Cardiac rehabilitation certification program, in Ribisl PM, et al: *Organizational Guidelines for Cardiac Rehabilitation Programs.* Winston-Salem, NC, Wake Forest Cardiac Rehabilitation Program, 1986.

Index

American College of Sports Medicine, 22, 171
Anger management training, 89-92
Angina pectoris (*see also* Pain), 28-29
    and work status, 142
Anxiety, 24, 68-69
    treatment of, 68-69
    on CCU, 68-69
Anxiety management training, 88-89
Assessment, psychologic, 21-39

Beck Depression Inventory, 25
Behavioral disturbances (*see* Personality disturbances)
Behavioral medicine, definition of, 2
Beta blockers, 118-128
    and anxiety reduction, 120-123
    properties of, 119
    psychologic effects, 120-126
    side effects of, 127
    and Type A behavior, 124-127
Biofeedback, 8-9
    assisted relaxation, 87-88
    blood pressure, 86-87
    cardiac arrhythmias, 88

CABGS (*see* Coronary artery bypass graft surgery)
Cardiac rehabilitation, certification of, 22, 169-170
    organization, 156-159
    patient admission criteria, 159-160
    programs, 155-171
Cardiac surgery (*see also* Coronary artery bypass graft surgery), 75-77
Compliance, 9-11

Index

Coronary artery bypass graft surgery (CABGS)
    and employment status, 133-143
    psychologic and social outcomes, 143-148
Coronary Care Unit (CCU), 24, 68-75
    transfer from, 75

Delirium
    and CABGS, 76-77
    on CCU, 72
    treatment, 72-73
Denial, 69-70
    treatment, 70
Depression, 25, 59-70
    treatment, 70
Diet, 4-6
Drill Book, 108-109

Emergency procedures, 168-169
Employment status, following CABGS, 133-138
    age, 133-138
    prediction of, 128-143
    socioeconomic status, 142-143
Exercise, 6-8, 161-162
    and anxiety, 54-56
    psychologic effects of, 53-65

Family conflicts, 74-75
Functional capacity, 29

Halstead-Reitan Aphasia Screening Test, 27
Hamilton Psychiatric Rating Scale, 26
Health care utilization, 29-30
Health status, perception of, 27-28
Hopkins Symptom Checklist, 25

Jacobson relaxation technique, 82-83
Jenkins Activity Survey, 31, 100-101

Life change, 30

Marlowe-Crowne Social Desirability Scale, 25
Marriage, 32-33
McGill Pain Questionnaire, 28
Medical assessment, 160-161
Medical status and employment, 141-142
Medication (*see also* Beta blockers), 29, 73-74

Index

Mini-Mental State, 26
Minnesota Multiphasic Personality Inventory (MMPI), 25
Multidisciplinary approach, 22, 166-167

National Exercise and Heart Disease Project, 60
Neuropsychologic assessment, 26-27
North Carolina Cardiac Rehabilitation Association, 170
Nutrition, 162-164

Pain (*see also* Angina pectoris), 28-29
Patient
    education, 167-168
    staffing, 166-167
Personality
    assessment of personality, 24-26
    disturbances, 71
    treatment, 71-72
Physical health, 27-28
Profile of Mood States, 25
Progress notes, 167-168
Progressive muscle relaxation, 82-84
Psychologic assessment, 21-39, 164-165

Recurrent Coronary Prevention Project, 104-112
Relapse and smoking, 45
Relaxation, 82-85
Russell Revised Wechsler Memory Scale, 26

Secondary prevention, 3
Sleep cycle defects, 74
Smoking, 3-4, 41-52
Smoking cessation, 42-44
    coping with, 45
    and relaxation, 46-47
    self-control strategies, 45-46
    sequelae of, 44-45
    and social support, 46
    and weight gain, 47-48
Social support, 32
    and smoking cessation, 46
Spielberger State-Trait Anxiety Questionnaire, 25
Structured interview, 30-31, 100

Taylor Manifest Anxiety Scale, 25
Trail Making Test, 27

Index

Type A behavior, 8, 30-31, 98-99
    modification of, 99-128
    pharmacologic treatment of, 117
Type A Self-Rating Inventory, 31

Vocational assessment, 165-166

Weight (*see* Diet)
Work, 33-34

Zung Self-Rating Depression Scale, 25